Community Programs for the Depressed Elderly: A Rehabilitation Approach

Community Programs for the Depressed Elderly: A Rehabilitation Approach

Ellen D. Taira
Editor

The Haworth Press
New York • London

Community Programs for the Depressed Elderly: A Rehabilitation Approach has also been published as *Physical & Occupational Therapy in Geriatrics,* Volume 5, Number 1, Fall 1986.

The Haworth Press, Inc., 12 West 32 Street, New York, NY 10001
EUROSPAN/Haworth, 3 Henrietta Street, London WC2E 8LU England

Library of Congress Cataloging in Publication Data

Community programs for the depressed elderly.

Includes bibliographies.
1. Depression in the aged. 2. Occupational therapy for the aged. 3. Community health services for the aged. I. Taira, Ellen D. [DNLM: 1. Community Mental Health Services—in old age. 2. Depression—in old age. 3. Depression—rehabilitation. 4. Occupational Therapy—in old age. WM 171 C7345]
RC537.5.C66 1987 362.2'0425 86-31956
ISBN 0-86656-644-9

Community Programs for the Depressed Elderly: A Rehabilitation Approach

Physical & Occupational Therapy in Geriatrics
Volume 5, Number 1

CONTENTS

Community Programs for the Depressed Elderly: A Rehabilitation Approach

FROM THE EDITOR

The papers in this first issue of volume five address a common theme: therapeutic intervention for the depressed older person. Depression is the most prevalent form of mental illness among older persons today (Eisdorfer, 1980). Loss of loved ones, financial security and functional independence contribute to feelings of emptiness, hopelessness and sadness that lead to depression. Despite this high incidence of mental illness, elderly persons are infrequent visitors to mental health clinics and receive only modest support from Medicare to pay for psychiatric services. Nevertheless, there are programs in community and institutional settings addressing the socialization and activity needs of the older person. The purpose of this issue of *Physical & Occupational Therapy in Geriatrics* is to familiarize practicing therapists with model programs for the depressed elderly.

These innovative programs were presented at the INTERNATIONAL SYMPOSIUM: OCCUPATIONAL THERAPY APPROACHES TO DEPRESSION IN OLDER PERSONS a conference held in New York City on July 11, 1985, sponsored by the Gerontology Special Interest Section of the American Occupational Therapy Association, Inc., and the programs in occupational therapy at Columbia University. The conference was held in conjunction with the XIII International Congress of Gerontology July 12 through 17th, also in New York. The six presenters from the symposium demonstrated the effectiveness of occupational therapy assessment and intervention with this underserved population.

All the presenters from the United States focused on elderly persons living in the community who were "at risk" of institutionalization due to affective illness. The occupational therapist's role was one of assessment, treatment and facilitation, respectively. The need to thoroughly assess patients to distinguish between depression and dementia and to accurately evaluate functional abilities was essential. The role of the occupational therapist in a home care setting where depression is a complication of chronic illness offers treatment intervention challenges to even the most experienced therapists.

The authors represent diverse backgrounds as occupational therapists. Model projects in countries where socialized forms of health care are available and programs for the elderly stress community living are described. Creating linkages between institutions and the community for the depressed elderly provides an especially appropriate role for occupational therapists with their focus on functional independence and activity.

The programs in Australia and Scotland have an especially important linkage component that may be unfamiliar to practicioners accustomed to a medical model rather than a holistic, preventive approach. The Danish program also offers an effective means of integrating a community resident into an institution by providing a "contact person" who follows the elderly person from home to nursing home and remains involved until the person has settled into institutional life.

This special issue would not have been possible without the assistance of Barbara Neuhaus, Acting Chair of the occupational therapy programs at Columbia University and Nancy Ellis, chairperson of the Gerontology Special Interest Section of the American Occupational Therapy Association. For their invaluable assistance editing these papers and providing input and support in the preparation of this issue, I should like to say a very special thank you.

EDT

REFERENCE

Eisdorfer, C., Cohen, D., Veith, R., (1980) The Psychopathology of Aging. Current Concepts. Upjohn.

Models for Treatment of Depression

Patricia Miller, MEd, OTR

The term depression is extremely complex, yet it is often used loosely. It can convey a vast spectrum of mood states from a blue Monday, which no life escapes, to a major depressive episode, otherwise called an affective disorder. This loose usage of the term can become problematic, as, for example, when a staff member of a long-term care facility observes a patient crying because of a disagreement with a roommate and then reports at a team meeeting that Mrs. X is "depressed." Is she? If so, where on the spectrum of depressive disorders does she belong? If not, the term was misused.

A broad psychiatric definition of depression is a disorder whose central feature is "a dysphoric mood . . . or loss of interest or pleasure in all or almost all ususal activities or pastimes" (Spitzer, 1980). There are three states of depression delineated for purposes of studying depression in the later years.

The first state is an uncomplicated grief reaction, which is often called reactive depression, and is the normal reaction to a loss. Symptoms such as poor appetite, weight loss and insomnia can occur along with tearfulness and varying degress of sadness. Morbid preoccupation with worthlessness and marked psychomotor retardation are uncommon. Thoughts of death are limited to feeling that he or she would have liked to have died with the loved one, rather than suicidal ruminations based on guilt and self-reproach. Late life reactive depressions are

---

Patricia Miller is Assistant Professor in Clinical Occupational Therapy, Columbia University and Consultant, Center for Geriatrics and Gerontology, Columbia University, New York.

Based on a presentation made at the International Symposium: Occupational Therapy Approaches to Depression in Older Adults, Pre-Congress Conference, XIII International Congress of Gerontology, July, 1985, Columbia University, New York.

very common because of the cumulative losses which can be superimposed upon each other. With advancing age and a clustering of losses, uncomplicated grief reactions can become complicated, leading to other types of depressive disorders.

The second depressive state is called a dysthymic disorder which was formerly known as neurotic depression. The disorder often begins without clear onset and may take a chronic course. Precipitating factors may or may not be identifiable. This disorder is usually not socially incapacitating and is non-psychotic. It is due to long-standing maladaptive patterns and is the result of unconscious conflicts.

The third depressive state is called major depressive episode, previously known as psychotic depression. Withdrawal from family and friends, loss of interest or pleasure in all activities, and at least four vegetative signs co-exist, and they are generally much more severe than in either of the first two states. Thoughts of death or suicide are common, and psychotic features may be present. In the depressed elderly, the presence of such symptoms as confusion, memory impairment and decreased levels of self-care may suggest dementia. This can very well be pseudodementia, not an organic condition. Making the differential diagnosis is extremely important, if depression is to be identified and treated.

It is generally agreed that regardless of what theory or school one adheres to, the heart of the therapeutic process is the relationship between the therapist and the patient. In fact, some studies indicate that individuals educated in a particular "school" are no more successful in effecting change than those people lacking formal training, who nevertheless are capable of demonstrating warmth and caring. If the therapist's attitude and personality are key variables in the change process, why bother learning theory? Theory serves as an immensely useful cognitive and perceptual map for assessment and treatment of patients (Michels, 1985).

This paper will address just a few theoretical models of depression and their application to practice. As there is no neat correlation between the theoretical formulations of depression and the three depressive states delineated earlier, the term depression will be used non-specifically. In discussing psychodynamic and cognitive theories, one observes that they are by no means mutually exclusive.

PSYCHODYNAMIC THEORIES

I—Freud's Model

Freud was the first major theorist to recognize the relationship between the emotional reactions to significant losses and the dynamics of depression (1957). Freud asserted that maladaptive childhood reaction patterns persist, often unconsciously, throughout life and are the cause of abnormal behavior. He also contrasted normal mourning and melancholia (now called major depression). Although loss is the common factor in both conditions, in melancholia loss is not accepted in a normal way. He postulated that severe depression or melancholia is due to aggression turned against the self. It is often caused by the loss of an ambivalently loved person, i.e., a person toward whom both feelings of love and hate co-existed. The feelings of hate that were once directed toward the lost person are now directed onto the self. A decrease in self-esteem, self-reproach, guilt and a need for punishment could culminate in suicide.

As occupational therapists, we are not trained to do psychoanalysis, nor would it ordinarily be the treatment of choice with a depressed elderly person. We can, however utilize psychodynamic theory as guidelines for assessment and treatment. For example, an in-depth history of the older person which includes facts and feelings about past life events may lead to insights regarding the person's present state of mind and attitudes regarding his or her future. Providing an opportunity for the patient to unburden himself by talking freely is an appropriate treatment approach based on this model. Developing a relationship of trust in which the patient's aggressive feelings can be gradually redirected and aiding the individual to gain insight into psychological conflicts while rebuilding self-esteem are also key components of this approach.

Case Example

A brief vignette to illustrate how psychodynamic theory works when used by an occupational therapist follows.

Assessment of a 78-year-old woman at a senior center,

(Mrs. G.) revealed depressive symptoms. She stated that she had no desire to participate in activities at the Center because she didn't get along well with people and that there wasn't too much she could do anymore. Upon further questioning, Mrs. G. talked about her preoccupation with her father's death. She regretted that she didn't tell her father she loved him before he died. She talked about her hospitalized sister, with whom she feels unable to communicate, although she visits her regularly. She stated that she is angry that she can't hear well enough to enjoy concerts; and because of painful knees, trips to museums have stopped.

The therapist noted this woman to be alert, very intelligent, highly negativistic and unkempt. She refused to participate in Center activities, but attended two to three times per week for the hot, noon-day meal. The occupational therapist worked with Mrs. G. individually for two sessions to establish trust and to allow her to unburden herself by talking. Mrs. G. then agreed to join a painting to music group. Toward the end of the painting session, each member of the group took turns interpreting their paintings to the other participants. Mrs. G. depicted three phases of her life in her drawing and explained to the group that the first section depicted her youth as a dancer, the second, her middle years of going to museums and concerts with friends. The third section, illustrating the present, was blank. With barely contained anger, she explained to the other members, "Nothing gives me pleasure anymore. I have so much pain!" Whereupon she picked up a piece of charcoal and scribbled lines in the blank section of her drawing.

At this point, another member who painted with great difficulty because of deformed, arthritic hands described her own drawing of a sunny, beach scene. She stated that the painting to music made her feel transported to the beach. Mrs. G. perceptively remarked that she needed to reveal her misery before she could move on to happier thoughts.

Several sessions later, Mrs. G. drew a picture of flowers depicting spring. In discussing the drawing with the group, she became aware of feeling guilty about enjoying the painting activity. "I really don't deserve to do this," she said sadly. In an impressive burst of insight a few minutes later, Mrs. G. said she realized that feeling guilty about a variety of things kept her from having a good time. The group members were supportive, telling Mrs. G. that they were glad she was a member of the painting group.

An expressive arts group served as a treatment strategy for applying psychodynamic theory. It encouraged self-expression and insight through imagery and association. For Mrs. G. it provided a channel for constructive redirection of aggressive feelings and an opportunity to reexperience pleasurable activity with peers and, to increase self-esteem.

II—Butler's Model

Robert Butler's theory of life review and his guidelines for life review therapy are psychoanalytically derived. Butler noted that "recovering important memories is a basic ingredient of the curative process in psychoanalysis and necessary for change" (Osgood, 1985). He states that the older years bring with it the mental process called life review. It is characterized by the return to consciousness of past experiences, especially unresolved conflicts and preoccupations with the death of others (Butler, 1982). Life review can then be considered "a natural form of self-analysis" (Osgood, p. 164).

Life review therapy, of which reminiscence is a part, can allow older people to express guilt, fear, grief and uneasiness along with a range of positive emotions.

Case Example

Occupational therapy for a 73-year-old depressed woman with osteoarthritis and diverticulitis, who was seen for home care, incorporated psychodynamic concepts and life review therapy in a program to increase functional ability and reduce depression. Mrs. B. claimed that she was old, weak, and ready to die. She remained in bed all day long and had insomnia at night. Her husband, an 80-year-old retired newspaper editor, was devoted to his wife and feared her institutionalization.

Treatment centered initially around writing down her thoughts, and, because Mrs. B. loved poetry, she tried to write poetically. Unresolved conflicts related to her mother and concerns about her relationship with her husband appeared in her writings. She began to look forward to sitting up in bed, and her tolerance for activity gradually increased. Self-care activities were slowly introduced and reinforced at each visit.

The occupational therapist began to include Mrs. B.'s husband in part of the therapy sessions as an adjunct therapist. With encouragement, they began to reminisce about some of their happier times together and to talk more directly of their hard times as well. Conversation between them, which was no longer a habit because of Mrs. B's prolonged, depressed withdrawal, became rivitalized. Completing an unfinished travel scrapbook, which included many family photos, became a prescribed activity for patient and husband to do together. After two months of twice weekly occupational therapy, Mrs. B. ambulated throughout her apartment with a walker, dressed herself, and showed a generally positive affect. Despite some continued complaints about not being able to do what she used to do, talk of wanting to die ceased and an interest in family and friends returned.

III—Bibring's Model

In the 1950's Edward Bibring, a psychoanalyst, described the mechanism of depression differently from Freud and his contribution has been widely recognized. Bibring formulated the mechanism of depression as the individual's shocking awareness of real or imaginary helplessness, which is accompanied by a loss of self-esteem. The depressed person sees himself as unable to live up to highly-valued (narcissistic) aspirations such as the wish to be worthy, and appreciated; to be strong, superior and secure; and to be good and loving (1961).

This model seems well-suited to the elderly person who does not necessarily reduce his standards in keeping with decreasing capacities, and, thus, becomes depressed.

Assessment and treatment approaches appropriate to this model include:

1. determine the conditions causing feelings of helplessness and hopelessness. To what extent are these feelings real or imaginary?
2. aid the patient in seeing his strengths and limitations in perspective, and,

3. encourage participation in meaningful activities in which strengths can be supported and enhanced, thereby increasing self-esteem.

Case Example

A 74-year-old director of a dancing school with a severe auto-immune disease was referred for occupational therapy in her home. Initial assessment revealed a very intelligent woman with symptoms of forgetfulness, short attention span, generalized weakness and dependency in most self-care activities except eating. Mrs. S. spoke of her difficulty in supervising the dance teachers and administering the school. She held meetings in her home at bedside, and became increasingly anxious and depressed in anticipation of the meetings. "I'm no good anymore. I can't remember. I've lost their respect."

Using Bibring's model, the therapist helped Mrs. S. put her strengths and limitations in perspective. By drawing a picture of the brain and showing Mrs. S. that her pathology was limited to the area of memory function, the patient was helped to acknowledge her remaining strength. The helplessness was no longer experienced as global once the pathology was isolated. Activities such as keeping a diary of administrative tasks to be delegated to Mrs. S's secretary helped relieve feelings of being out of control. Making a list of remaining strengths and how to use them with teachers and students was discussed and practiced. For example, although Mrs. S. had difficulty remembering names, she could talk about her philosophy of dance in an inspirational way. She was encouraged to do so while receiving support for releasing the reins in her areas of diminishing abilities. Mrs. S. died three months from the start of occupational therapy. Friends, colleagues and the therapist observed Mrs. S. to be less self-depreciatory and more relaxed and communicative in her last weeks of life.

A COGNITIVE THEORY

Moving from the psychodynamic theories to a cognitive paradigm, Aaron Beck delineated three cognitive patterns which can be identified in varying degrees in most depressive disorders.

In the first pattern, the patient consistently interprets his interaction with his environment as representing defeat and deprivation. In the second, he views himself in a negative way: deficient, inadequate or unworthy. The third pattern consists of viewing the future negatively. He anticipates that his suffering will continue indefinitely. This negative view of the world, the self and the future leads to a depressed mood, paralysis of will, increased dependency, avoidance and suicidal wishes (Beck, 1967).

Beck's formulations have direct application to our goals of breaking the inactivity cycle, increasing motivation and functional ability. First, by knowing an individual's cognition, Beck explains, "one can predict his motivation or lack of it" (p. 263). "Second, by changing his cognition one can change his motivation. The loss of motivation may be viewed as the result of the patient's hopelessness and pessimism; as long as he expects a negative outcome from any course of action, he is stripped of any internal stimulation to do anything about it. It becomes necessary to persuade the depressed person that a positive outcome may result from a particular endeavor" (p. 264).

Older people, particularly those who are depressed, may have the same ageist attitudes as the rest of society. "I'm too old." "Why bother with me?" "That's for young people." These are familiar refrains. The relatively younger therapist must examine his or her own attitudes toward aging and the aged, and assist the older person to view himself and his relationship to the environment in a more positive way. Confronting the ageist attitudes of society with which the patient identifies and kindly disagreeing with them helps the depressed person to feel less unworthy and more hopeful.

At the same time, the pervasive feelings of helplessness and hopelessness, the increased dependency and inactivity must be explained to the patient as part of the depressive disorder. When patients are helped to recognize and understand the negative cycle that develops from feeling helpless, to inactivity, to feeling more helpless, to increased inactivity, it is a step toward breaking that cycle. Feelings of being inept, inadequate and undesirable contribute to increased dependency. The patient feels that the task of reversing his depression is insurmountable. The therapist can meet the patient's dependency needs by stating, "We will work on breaking this inactivity cycle together." A working alliance between therapist and patient must be developed to enable the patient to take the first steps toward renewed health.

CONCLUSION

In summary, psychodynamic and cognitive models of depression are just a few of the many models which can be used as guidelines for assessment and treatment. Goals of all the models described are reducing the feelings of helplessness and hopelessness and rebuilding self-esteem.

The case for a single theoretical approach is argued in terms of having a ready-made set of assumptions, concepts, strategies and research potential. However, the later years of life are complex, requiring an application of broad and varied strategies and methods. In clinical practice, this therapist has drawn both consciously and automatically from the treatment approaches of several schools to meet the multiple and varied needs of older patients. These treatment strategies integrate theoretical models that have relevance to a particular person, in a particular setting, at a particular time. Whether a single or an eclectic theoretical approach is utilized, non-specific curative factors common to all effective treatment models must be in effect: acceptance, non-possessive warmth, genuineness, hope, and accurate empathy.

REFERENCES

Beck, Aaron, *Depression—Clinical, Experimental and Theoretical Aspects,* Harper and Row, New York, 1967.

Bibring, Edward, "The Mechanism of Depression," *Affective Disorders, Psychoanalytic Contributions to their Study,* Edited by Phyllis Greenacre, Intern'tl Univ. Press, N.Y., 1961.

Butler, R. and Lewis, M. *Aging and Mental Health—Positive Psychosocial and Biomedical Approaches,* 3rd Ed., CV Mosby, Co., 1982.

Freud, Sigmund, "Mourning and Melancholia," *The Complete Psychological Works of Sigmund Freud,* Vol. XIV, Hogarth Press, London, 1957.

Michels, Robert, "The Meaning of Theory in Psychiatric Practice," guest speaker, Westchester Psychoanalytic Institute annual dinner meeting, May, 1985.

Osgood, Nancy, *Suicide in the Elderly—A Practitioner's Guide to Diagnosis and Mental Health Intervention,* Aspen Systems Corp., 1985.

Spitzer, Robert, *Diagnostic and Statistical Manual of Mental Disorders,* DSM, III, 3rd edition, American Psychiatric Assoc., Washington, D.C., 1980.

Occupational Therapy Assessment for Older Adults With Depression: Asking the Right Questions

Joan C. Rogers, PhD, OTR

ABSTRACT. Occupational performance is posited to be a multifaceted construct involving self-perceptions of competence, habits of daily living, skills of daily living, and occupational performance components. This article describes the assessment of occupational performance in older adults with depression. The questions guiding the assessment are delineated, the appropriate data-gathering methodologies are identified, the characteristic yield obtained from depressed older adults is described, and the occupational diagnosis is illustrated.

The initial contact between two individuals is oriented toward getting acquainted with the other individual. In the professional relationship, the professional seeks to understand the patient in terms of the unique helping skills that he or she possesses. The patient, on the other hand, tries to understand the kind of help that is available from the helper. The process of getting acquainted is called the assessment. Unlike informal human interactions, the assessment is highly focused and structured. The professional directs the development of the helping relationship and strives to give and elicit salient information as economically as possible.

The purpose of the occupational therapy assessment is to

Joan C. Rogers is Professor of Occupational Therapy and Assistant Professor of Psychiatry, Geriatric Psychiatry and Behavioral Neurology Module, Western Psychiatric Institute and Clinic, 3811 O'Hara Street, University of Pittsburgh, Pittsburgh, PA 15213.

This paper is based on a presentation made at the International Symposium: Occupational Therapy Approaches to Depression in Older Adults, Pre-Congress Conference, XIII International Congress of Gerontology, July, 1985, Columbia University, New York.

elucidate the occupational nature of patients so that a therapeutic regimen to resolve or alleviate occupational performance dysfunctions or sharpen occupational performance can be developed and implemented. The assessment process, which aims at assisting the therapist to know the patient and the patient to understand occupational therapy services, is guided by four key questions: (1) What are the patient's perceptions of competence in occupational performance? (2) What are the paitent's habits of daily living? (3) What are the patient's skills in daily living? (4) What factors facilitate or hinder occupational performance? Each question explores a different facet of occupational functioning. Each facet contributes to the totality of occupational performance. The therapist's diagnostic expertise is exhibited in apprehending each facet uniquely and merging them into a cohesive theory to explain the patient's occupational functioning. Professional skill is evidenced in exploring each question in a sensitive and humanizing manner and establishing an effective working alliance between the therapist and patient.

In this article, the occupational therapy assessment is described in relation to the older adult with depression. Since depression is the most common affective disorder experienced by persons over age 65, affecting about 10 percent of this population (Blazer, 1982), any therapist working with this age group needs to be able to assess the impact of depression on occupational functioning. The specific objectives of the article are to: delineate the key questions guiding the assessment, identify the data-gathering methodology appropriate for answering each question, describe the typical yield for each question obtained from depressed older adults, and illustrate the process of formulating an occupational diagnosis.

SELF-PERCEPTIONS

Self-perceptions of competence refers to the patient's *beliefs* about his or her occupational performance. Occupational performance spans the gamut of self-care, home management, work, and leisure occupations. Tasks included in the self-care category are feeding, dressing, hygiene, grooming, bathing and mobility. Home management may be broken down into planning and preparing meals, shopping, housekeeping and housecleaning, gardening, doing home repairs, managing money, and using the telephone. Work and leisure activities are highly individualized. For each occupational performance category, the therapist is interested in ascertaining the patient's beliefs about the tasks that he or she can do.

Data about self-perceptions are obtained through self-report and self-rating. The therapist asks the patient questions about his or her abilities. Although some questions may be presented in written form, an interviewing procedure predominates. The questions are usually very specific rather than general. For example, "Can you balance your checkbook?" in contrast to "What can you do?" For tasks for which competence is expressed, further inquiry focuses on the ease of task performance. The therapist is interested in grouping tasks into those that can be accomplished with ease and with difficulty. When inabilities are stated or implied, questioning centers on the perceived reasons for dysfunction.

Self-perceptions of competence in occupational tasks are examined to gain knowledge of how the patient sees his or her abilities. Normally, humans do not attempt to do things unless they feel that they have a chance of being successful. Self-perceptions are therefore predictive of what a patient does or will do. When the patient's perceptions of competence are in agreement with his or her actual performance skills, the patient possesses insight into his or her occupational functioning. By comparing the patient's self-perceptions with his or her skill, the therapist can ascertain the areas and extent of agreement and disagreement.

Older adults with depression typically see themselves as unable rather than able. They provide a long list of tasks they are unable to do at all or are unable to do to their own satisfaction. Negative ratings of tasks performance are often accompanied by expressions of worthlessness, helplessness, and hopelessness. Task dysfunction is often attributed to fatigue, a lack of energy, and inability to think or concentrate, or vague illness; less commonly to emotional or motivational factors. As affective improvement occurs, perceptions of competence and incompetence become more reality based, that is to say they conform to the patient's skill level.

HABITS

Habits of daily living refers to tasks that an individual performs on a *routine* basis or *performed in the past* but is no longer doing. Rather than inquiring about tasks that the patient thinks he or she can do, questioning is oriented toward what the patient actually does. The intent is to describe what the person's day-by-day life is like. The therapist seeks to understand how the patient actually spends time. The appraisal includes the ability to coordinate daily life tasks into an effective life-style as well as to accomplish the necessary activities. The evaluation of habits provides a portrait of how effectively time is allocated for self-care, home management, leisure, and work occupations.

The primary data-gathering methodology for habit evaluation is questioning. As with the evaluation of self-perceptions, questioning may be done through interviews or questionnaires. Commonly, these data-gathering methods are used in a complementary fashion. A written questionnaire is completed and its content is enriched when it is discussed with the therapist.

Information about daily living habits is generally obtained from the patient and a knowledgeable informant. Family members, caregivers, and neighbors are potential sources of information. In the case of patients residing in institutional settings or hospitalized, nursing staff can also provide data about self-care routines. Questioning includes consideration of the help received from others as well as the patient's attitudes toward receiving help and caregivers' attitudes toward giving it.

In addition to eliciting information, the therapist must also appraise the validity of the information received. Validity deals with the extent to which the information obtained about habit patterns corresponds to what the patient actually does or did. Regardless of the source of the information, data about habits should agree, since the same thing is being appraised. Data about daily living habits may fail to correspond to those habits for numerous reasons. For example, a patient who is acutely depressed may accentuate inabilities to impress upon the therapist the seriousness of his or her condition or to bolster the chance of receiving maximum aid. A caregiver who only sees the patient for 4 hours over the weekend may not know enough about the patient to give an accurate report of habit patterns. The possibility of error arising from reporting bias, informant ignorance, and other sources must be weighed by the therapist before data are accepted as valid indicators.

The evaluation of habits extends beyond an investigation of current status to past status. Habits have a developmental nature. They are learned over time. With the exception of personal self-care tasks, such as feeding and dressing, which must be accomplished in some manner by all humans, habits are singular for each individual. Not all older adults have learned how to make beds or write checks. The therapist is interested in ascertaining the skills that have been learned, since this knowledge is critical for formulating the occupational therapy diagnosis. An elderly widower who has never done laundry, would be viewed differently than one who has. In the former case, the problem is that of initial skill learning or locating someone to do the laundry. In the latter case, skill disuse or breakdown must be entertained.

In addition to documenting the accumulation of learned skills, the therapist is also interested in tracing the emergence of occupational performance dysfunction associated with depression. As previously implied, the negative self-perceptions of occupational performance are generally accompanied by a severe deterioration of habits. This deterioration is often in sharp contrast to a successful and effective occupational history. Current habit patterns are laid against pre-episodic or pre-illness patterns to ascertain the areas affected by change as well as the amount, rate, and sequence of change. Change may be abrupt or gradual extending over months or years. A loss of interest in activities that were previously stimulating is apparent. Activities outside the home may be those first affected. Productivity is decreased. Daily life is characterized by long periods of inactivity, negligible structure, and minimal obligated time. Futurity is constricted and the ability to plan is almost non-existent. Habit deterioration involves a lowering of personal and/or socially acceptable standards. This leads to unacceptable behavior such as sloppy work, unkempt appearance, and eventual relinquishment of task responsibility. Habit deterioration characteristic of depression does not involve inappropriate behaviors such as self-exposure or incontinence. As a result of habit breakdown, daily life occupations are now supervised by or done by others. This "external control" reinforces a sense of incompetence and inadequacy. Despite dependence on others, however, there is generally no real sense of connectedness to them. Caregivers typically sense that depressed patients can do more for themselves than they are doing and may resent this dependency. Patients, on the other hand, simply feel they cannot manage and need help. With affective improvements, habits are reconstituted, productivity is increased, and personal control is resumed.

SKILL

While self-perceptions of competence refers to beliefs about occupational performance and habits of daily living routines, skill refers to the older adult's *ability to perform tasks.* To obtain information about an individual's skill, the skill must be observed. This is achieved through performance testing in actual or simulated living, playing, and working environments. In effect, the therapist asks the patient to demonstrate his or her ability to do a wide range of occupational tasks.

When performance testing takes place in the environment where the individual actually performs (home, workplace, etc.), as occurs in home health and industry, testing takes advantage of the individual's familiarity with the task environment. In preparing a meal in one's kitchen, for example, past experience enables one to know how to operate the stove and where to find the proper ingredients. Dysfunction due to unfamiliarity can be readily appreciated by anyone who has tried to cook in someone else's kitchen! When performance testing is done in the actual task environment, it is reasonable to assume that the individual is familiar with the location and use of tools, equipment, and materials, unless there has been a recent relocation. This is *NOT* a reasonable assumption when the task environment is simulated.

In addition to familiarity, performance testing in the actual task environment allows the therapist to take into account the manner in which the patient interacts with the environment.

The impaired older adult, for example, needs to get in and out of his or her bathtub safely, not just any bathtub. Ascertaining the mere presence of a bathtub safety rail through questioning is inadequate, since it tells the therapist nothing about the patient's use of that equipment. By observing the patient transferring into and out of the bathtub, the therapist can judge the efficiency and safety of performance.

The qualities of familiarity and person-environment interaction are particularly important to be aware of in the evaluation of older adults because they are more dependent on the environment than younger adults. Their habit structures are tied to particular pieces of equipment in particular settings and it becomes difficult to adapt to newness and novelty. At the same time, when the accumulation of disease-related and age-related impairments reduce personal adaptability, the environment can often be modified to enhance occupational performance.

While evaluation in the actual task environment is generally preferable, performance testing in simulated clinical settings is more common. When testing is carried out under contrived conditions, the therapist must accommodate for unfamiliarity and for the gaps between the actual and simulated tasks environments. To accommodate for a lack of familiarity, the older patient must be systematically oriented to the task environment by the examiner prior to testing. To accommodate for incongruity between the actual and simulated situation, the simulation must meet the specifications of the actual environment as much as possible. This reduces the degree of extrapolation from performance under simulated circumstances to actual conditions.

Clinical simulations of normal living environments often embody ideal task conditions. Equipment and materials are arranged to accommodate reduced manual dexterity, impaired short term memory, wheelchairs and the like. Thus, in some instances, the incongruity between the actual and contrived task environments becomes an advantage rather than a disadvantage. Performance in the contrived environment that is not replicated in the actual environment suggests that environmental modifications may resolve the occupational performance dysfunction.

Performance testing furnishes vital information about

occupational performance capabilities. When an individual becomes emotionally, mentally, or physically impaired, assistance with daily living tasks is often provided. With the passage of time, individuals may become unsure about their performance ability. When asked if they can do a task, they may respond, "I don't know," or "I think I can, but I haven't done it in a while," or "My daughter does that for me now, I don't have to." Such responses make questioning a problematic methodology for obtaining information about skill. Observation of task performance allows the therapist to formulate a list, similar to those constructed by the patient and informants, of tasks the patient can do with ease, and hence independently, and those that can be done with difficulty or not at all, and hence require assistance and/or training.

Characteristically, depressed older adults exhibit few, if any, skill dysfunctions. Once they have been cajoled to do something, their performance may be slow, and even automatic, but there is no real difficulty completing familiar tasks. Due to diurnal mood variation, performance is generally better in the afternoon than morning. On occasion, the pace of task performance is accelerated rather than retarded. Agitation may be apparent. It is not uncommon for patients to do tasks that they have previously stated that they could not do. Patients usually seem to be unaware of this contradiction. When asked about the discrepancy, they often attribute skill to chance external factors or discount it. Despite good or acceptable performance, patients may be neutral or even negative about their performance or the end product. There is an inability to experience the pleasure of achievement. If skill dysfunctions are identified in depressed older adults, they are usually sporadic. Performance is variable rather than consistently poor. Alternatively, the deficit may be induced by something other than depression. Improvement in affective status is discernible in speed of task performance and pleasure in achievement.

In view of the indecision that may accompany task selection in depressed individuals, it is generally preferable to conduct the performance test in a manner that negates decision-making regarding task selection, except when decision-making is under scrutiny. For example, the performance test is approached by saying, "Show me how you make the bed," rather than "Will you show me how you make the bed?" or "These are the things that I would like you to do. Where would you like to begin." If the patient is particularly regressed at the time of assessment, naturalistic observation during the normal routine time of the activity may be substituted for performance testing. For example, the patient may be observed doing morning care routines upon rising. Naturalistic observation may also be done when the patient is confused or as a matter of convenience.

OCCUPATIONAL PERFORMANCE COMPONENTS

To plan a course of treatment, it is often helpful to understand the factor or factors that hinder and facilitate task performance. These factors are called occupational performance components. Occupational performance components may be biological, psychological, or social in nature. Functional vision and postural balance are examples of biological components. Memory, judgement, and motivation are illustrative of psychological components. Factors outside the person, such as social attitudes and architectural barriers, represent social components.

More often than not, the older adult referred to occupational therapy has multiple medical conditions rather than just a singular diagnosis. The older patient with depression may also have osteoarthritis, cataracts, hiatal hernia, and diabetes. Depression may co-exist with dementia. These multisystem problems often translate into multifactoral impairments that span the biopsychosocial components of occupational performance. Thus, when evaluating a depressed older adult it is hazardous to focus only on the psychosocial components of occupational performance and neglect the biological components simply because depression is the precipitating reason for the occupational therapy referral.

The occupational performance components are generally evaluated by clinical observations, procedures and instruments, and standardized tests. Goniometry, manual muscle testing and sensory testing are examples of evaluations tapping the biological components. Mental status, mood, and perceptual tests probe psychological components. Inventories examining role participation and attitudinal scales appraising caregiver burden reflect the social components. Evaluations of component functions done by other professionals are useful adjuncts to the occupational therapy evaluations.

For depressed older adults, rating scales, such as the Geriatric Depression Scale (Yesavage et al., 1980), the Self-Rating Depression Scale (Zung, 1965), the Depression Inventory (Beck, 1961), and the Hamilton Depression Rating Scale (Hamilton, 1967) may be used to confirm or supplement mood observations made in conjunction with the evaluation of habits, skills, and self-perceptions of competence. Characteristically, depressed patients acknowledge physiological disturbances such as constipation, rapid heart beat, and fatigue, along with decreases in sleep, appetite and sexual interest. Weight loss may also be noted. Subjectively, patients feel "blue," sad, depressed, and may admit to crying spells. Psychomotor disturbances of restlessness and retardation and an inability to do ordinary things are also recognized. Expected ideational disturbances include confusion, emptiness, hopelessness, indecision, irritability, dissatisfaction, personal devaluation, and suicidal thoughts (Verwoerdt, 1976).

SEQUENCE OF ASSESSING OCCUPATIONAL PERFORMANCE

The facets of occupational performance that are generally evaluated first are self-perceptions and habits. As previously discussed, these facets rely on questioning. The therapist initially encourages patients to talk about themselves in a focused way. At some point, the therapist seeks to corroborate the data obtained from patients about daily living habits with knowledgeable informants.

Following the questioning process, the patient is asked to demonstrate skill in daily living activities. Simultaneously, the therapist screens for assets and deficits in the components of occupational performance. When necessary, deficit components are subsequently evaluated in-depth. The occupational therapy assessment as described in this article is outlined in Figure 1.

CASE ILLUSTRATION

To make the four facets of occupational performance more meaningful, each will be illustrated in regard to Mrs. G., who is an 83-year-old woman of Italian heritage. She was brought to the hospital by Mrs. M., a daughter-in-law, because of withdrawal and a decreased ability to care for herself. Mrs. G. indicated "all I want to do is sleep and never wake up again." Although she seems to welcome death, she had made no suicide attempts and verbalized no efforts directed toward this end. Her husband (a plumber), of 69 years died 18 months ago after an extended illness. Her two sons, ages 66 and 67, died suddenly within 2 weeks of each other about 4 months ago. Her 4 daughters reside out-of-state and rarely visit their mother because of a lack of money. There is frequent telephone and written communication and each daughter has invited Mrs. G. to live with her. Mrs. G. feels that she has had relatively good health all her adult life. There is no history of psychiatric illness in the family. Mrs. G. has degenerative joint disease, lens implants in both eyes secondary to cataracts, and macular degeneration in the right eye. She lives alone in the house where she raised her children. This is a 10 room tri-level suburban house with bathrooms on the first (basement) and third (bedrooms) levels.

Self-Perceptions

In response to direct questioning, Mrs. G. indicated that she could feed herself but had difficulty chewing because of loose dentures. She commented that she had no appetite for food, but felt that she had maintained her weight over the past two years. (The waist of her slacks was hanging on her hips.) She indicated that she had no problems dressing herself. She takes a sponge bath because she is afraid of falling in the bathtub. (An unpleasant body odor was obvious.) Mrs. G. reported that she falls about once per month, but that she has never hurt herself. She said that she was able to climb stairs (about 10) to the bathroom and that she could get there "on time." She gets up at least twice each night to urinate. She stated that she was accustomed to going to the beauty parlor to have her hair done but had no way to get there now

Figure 1

OCCUPATIONAL THERAPY ASSESSMENT OF OLDER ADULT WITH DEPRESSION

FACET OF OCCUPATIONAL PERFORMANCE	Self-perceptions of Competence
DEFINITION	Patient's beliefs about his/her occupational performance
GUIDING QUESTIONS	What do you think you can do?
DATA-GATHERING METHODOLOGY	Questioning the patient
TYPICAL RESPONSE FOR DEPRESSED OLDER ADULTS	° Perceptions of incompetence ° Incompetence attributed to fatigue, lack of energy, inability to concentrate, or vague illness ° With affective improvement, perceptions conform to skill level
THERAPIST YIELD	° Description of tasks patient believes he/she can do easily, with difficulty, and not at all ° Index predictive of habits ° Index for detecting change over time ° Index of patient's insight into occupational functioning when self-perceptions and skills are compared ° Index of occupational performance components influencing performance and requiring further evaluation

FACET OF OCCUPATIONAL PERFORMANCE	Skill
DEFINITION	Ability to perform tasks
GUIDING QUESTIONS	What can you do?
DATA-GATHERING METHODOLOGY	Performance testing Naturalistic observation

Figure 1 (Continued)

FACET OF OCCUPATIONAL PERFORMANCE	Skill
TYPICAL RESPONSE FOR DEPRESSED OLDER ADULTS	° Adequate or better completion of familiar tasks; on occasion performance is variable ° Improved performance in afternoon ° Pace is usually slow but may be accelerated and agitation may be present ° Performance appears automatic and labored ° Incapacity for enjoyment ° With affective improvement, normal activity pace is resumed, performance reflects spontaneity and is consistent throughout the day, and pleasure is derived from activity
THERAPIST YIELD	° Description of patient's maximum performance capability ° Index of degree of occupational dysfunction when compared with habits ° Index of detecting change over time ° Index of occupational performance components influencing performance and requiring further evaluation

FACET OF OCCUPATIONAL PERFORMANCE	Habits of Daily Living
DEFINITION	Tasks the patient performs routinely or performed in the past but is no longer doing
GUIDING QUESTIONS	What do you do? What have you done?
DATA-GATHERING METHODOLOGY	Questioning the patient and knowledgeable informants
TYPICAL RESPONSE FOR DEPRESSED OLDER ADULT	° Abrupt or gradual loss of interest in activities ° Deterioration of habits involving a lowering of standards and relinquishment of task responsibility

Figure 1 (Continued)

FACET OF OCCUPATIONAL PERFORMANCE	Habits of Daily Living
	° Increase in unstructured and unobligated time ° Constricted view of future and contingent lack of planfulness ° With affective improvement, habits are reconstituted
THERAPIST YIELD	° Description of current occupational status and daily life ° Occupational history documenting skills, the patient's highest level of functioning, and the advent and rate of occupational dysfunction ° Standard for determining whether current occupational functioning reflects skill breakdown, disuse, or need for initial skill learning ° Indices of caregiver attitudes toward giving help and patient attitudes toward receiving help ° Index for detecting change over time ° Index of informant accuracy and bias when information from data sources and methodologies are compared ° Index of occupational performance components influencing performance and requiring further evaluation

FACET OF OCCUPATIONAL PERFORANCE	Occupational Performance Components
DEFINITION	Biological, psychological and social components of occupational performance
GUIDING QUESTIONS	What factors promote and hinder the performance of a task?
DATA-GATHERING METHODOLOGY	° Screened for simultaneously with evaluation of self-perception habits and skills ° Evaluated using formal and informal observation, questioning and testing

Figure 1 (Continued)

FACET OF OCCUPATIONAL PERFORMANCE	Occupational Performance Components
TYPICAL RESPONSE FOR DEPRESSED OLDER ADULTS	° Subjective feelings of depression, sadness; crying spells are common ° Physiological disorders of constipation, rapid heart beat, fatigue, and losses of sleep, appetite and sexual desire; acknowledgment of weight loss ° Awareness of restlessness and/or retardation of action and an inability to do ordinary daily tasks ° Expressions of confusion, emptiness, hopelessness, indecision, irritability, dissatisfaction, personal devaluation, and suicidal thoughts
THERAPIST YIELD	° Multifactorial description of patient's strength and weaknesses and their impact on occupational performance ° Indepth description of mood

and could not do her own hair. (Her hair was neatly combed but unstyled.) She indicated that she took care of her own fingernails and toenails and oral hygiene. (Fingernails were trimmed; toenails were unusually long.) She is not taking any regular medication. She felt that she was unable to do anything around the house because "I am not feeling well . . . I'm sick . . . I don't know what is wrong . . . I can't do anything . . . I am old . . . I am useless . . . take me to the cemetery, I want to be with my husband." When asked about her leisure skills, she replied, "I used to sew, knit, crochet, embroider, read. Now, I don't do anything. I sleep and I can't even do that well anymore." In response to further probes about her ability to continue her leisure pastimes she said, "It has been a long time. I don't know. I can't read. I can read, but I can't remember what I read."

Habits

Mrs. G. has been a homemaker all her life. She spoke with pride about "raising 6 beautiful children," "being an accomplished seamstress," "keeping a clean house," and "growing her own vegetables and flowers." According to Mrs. M.,

> Mrs. G. was a fastidious housekeeper. She stopped going to school while in the fourth grade to take care of her 5 brothers and sisters, all of whom are deceased. She always made her own clothes; most of the clothes for her children; and special clothing, such as Communion outfits, for her 16 grandchildren. She has not sewed for over 3 years—"since my husband got sick."

Mrs. G. never learned how to drive a car or use public transportation. Since her husband's death, her daughter-in-law (whom she always refers to as my son's wife), has taken her food shopping and for medical appointments. Mrs. G. is aware of local transportation for seniors, but feels that her family should take care of her, since she always took care of them. Mrs. M. also manages Mrs. G.'s finances, a task previously done by Mr. G. Mrs. G. was accustomed to walking regularly to the beauty parlor and to church every morning. She now has her hair done infrequently and has stopped attending church. A neighbor is paid to mow the grass and do odd jobs. Mrs. G. was never active in parent, social, or civic groups, since her husband "did these things." Her friends, who were her neighbors, have died, moved away, or become ill. She has no one whom she regards as a friend. Mrs. G. describes herself as having "lived for my husband and my family." She has always had little interest in watching television, except for the news.

Mrs. G.'s performance began to deteriorate after her husband's death. She stopped tending the garden and routine housecleaning was no longer done adequately. Thinking that his mother was no longer able to do the housekeeping, the eldest son paid for a housekeeper one day per week, and gave this service to his mother as a gift. Although Mrs. G. allowed the housekeeper to clean the house, change the bed, and do the laundry, she was very angry with her son for "doing this to her" and refused to speak to her son or the housekeeper. This situation was unresolved when her son died. Mrs. G. gradually increased her use of prepared foods (TV dinners), most of which went uneaten. Mrs. M. started fixing meals for

Mrs. G. 3 months ago. Her food intake has not improved and she has lost about 60 pounds over the past 2 years. She appears thin and frail.

Immediately prior to hospitilization, Mrs. G. was still getting up at her usual time, 5:30 A.M. After making and drinking a cup of instant coffee, she would spend the day sitting, staring out of the window. Previously, she had done housekeeping chores in the morning and food shopping, yardwork, or handwork in the afternoon. She generally retired at 9:30 or 10:00 P.M. and maintains this as her bedtime. She has not put on street clothes since her son's funeral 4 months ago and has not been out of the house since then. She wears the same housecoat night and day and only changes it when the housekeeper insists. Neither Mrs. M. nor the housekeeper have been successful in persuading her to bathe.

As a recent widow, and one who has her own mother to look after, Mrs. M. (age 60) indicated that she could not continue to give daily care to her mother-in-law. Mrs. M. works part-time as a cashier in a supermarket. She feels that she is under constant stress because of the "orders" that she receives from the 4 daughters regarding their mother. The family is very angry at Mrs. M. for bringing Mrs. G. to a psychiatric hospital. Mrs. M. is the only person actively caring for Mrs. G. Mrs. M. is willing to give some care for Mrs. G., but feels that Mrs. G. can do more for herself and is taking advantage of her. Mrs. M. described her relationship with Mrs. G. as "OK," "cordial," "no real problems," but not "warm." Mrs. M. was unaware of any falls by Mrs. G.

Skill

Mrs. G. was observed upon rising as she bathed, washed and combed her hair, dressed, ate breakfast, and did oral hygiene. She completed these tasks independently and acceptably, although no attempt was made to style her hair, even when encouraged to do so. She did use the shower and the shower chair and only ate soft foods. When complimented about her appearance, she was unresponsive. She filed her fingernails upon request, but refused to do her toenails. Because of long toenails, she is unable to put shoes on and hence wears open-toed slippers. She agreed to have the podiatrist cut her toenails. She used her hands to push down on the chair armrests or on her thighs to assist in rising from a seated position. When ascending stairs, she used a reciprocal gait; when descending, she put two feet on each step. Hand railings were used and she watched where each foot was placed. Balance was adequate with these procedures. She was short of breathe after climbing 7 stairs and asked to rest before continuing. Tasks were done at a slow even pace.

Mrs. G. did a variety of light and heavy housekeeping chores—making a bed, fixing a hot lunch requiring the use of the range and oven, washing dishes, sorting and doing laundry, shopping for food, making purchases, mending a hem, vacuuming, dusting, using the telephone to request information, cleaning the refrigerator, writing out checks for utility payments, and balancing a checkbook. Mrs. G. was oriented to the location of equipment and tools. She did not request assistance in equipment usage. No help was given and none was needed. She sequenced and organized tasks effectively and completed all tasks adequately and safely. She was hesitant about using the stove and range. Since she was not used to cooking with electricity, she watched "things closer, so that they will not burn." Mrs. G. planned, sewed (on the machine), and stuffed a pillow. She attributed difficulty in getting the seam width even and wide enough to visual impairment. She self-corrected all errors. Mrs. G. refused to take the pillow with her saying, "I don't like it." As the session progressed, she kept repeating "This is silly . . . This is stupid . . . I can do all these things."

Occupational Performance Components

Fine-Motor skills and mobility appear to be most influenced by reductions in visual acuity. Mrs. G. is aware of the need to take safety precautions and does so routinely. Moderate lower extremity weakness was suggested by a score of 42 seconds on the "Timed Stands" Test (Csuka and McCarty, 1985), which is double the mean score for her age. On the Performance-Oriented Assessment of Mobility Problems (Tinetti, 1986), adaptive responses were indicated on the following tests in addition to use of arms in rising from a chair—standing with eyes closed and turning (needed to hold onto objects), when nudged on the sternum (moved feet but balance maintained), standing on one leg, back extension, and reaching up (loss of balance). No cognitive deficit was detected with the Mini-Mental State Examination (Folstein, Folstein, and McHugh, 1975), as concluded from a score of 30, which is the maximum possible. Mrs. G. obtained a score of 53 on the Beck (1961) Depression Inventory suggesting severe depression. As reported by both Mrs. G. and Mrs. M., Mrs. G.'s bathtub does not have safety rails or mats and there is no shower in the house. There are railings on the indoor but not the outdoor stairs. Lighting throughout is described as dark. Mrs. G. indicated that she wants to stay in her own home because if she went to live with one of her children, she would have to make a choice and this would hurt someone.

Descriptive Occupational Diagnosis

Mrs. G. has had a satisfactory and satisfying career as a homemaker for a family of 7. Disruption of her daily routine began about 3 years ago when her husband became ill and was manifested in a complete termination of sewing. She had previously spent considerable time engaged in sewing, found it enjoyable, and took pleasure in making things for herself and her family. Additional activity restrictions occurred at the time of her husband's death about 18 months ago, when her standards for home and yard work began to decline. With the exception of nutritional intake, personal self-care was maintained fairly adequately until the death of her two sons about 4 months ago. At this time, there were decremental changes in cleanliness and appearance and Mrs. G. became essentially homebound. Conflict with the eldest son regarding his provision of homemaker assistance remained unresolved at the time of his death.

Although Mrs. G. feels that her illness prevents her from doing household chores, she demonstrated the skill and endurance needed for light and heavy homemaking tasks. Concentration, problem-solving, and judgement were adequate for task demands. Despite life-long dependency in money management, she was able to write out checks and balance a checking account accurately. Activity pace although slow did not interfere substantively with task performance. Performance standards were acceptable. Completion of a sewing project appeared to elicit no pleasure. Perceptions of adequacy in dressing, toileting, oral hygiene, and finger nail care were confirmed by performance testing, as were problems in eating due to ill-fitting dentures and bathing due to fear of falling. Having never learned to drive or use public services, she is dependent on her daughter-in-law for transportation. Mrs. G. cites a lack of transportation to get to the hairdresser as the reason for her messy hair. History of falling remains unconfirmed. However, Mrs. G. exhibited shortness of breathe upon exertion, used available safety equipment, exercised appropriate precautions when moving, has confirmed lower extremity weakness and problems maintaining balance in test situations, complains of being unable to see where she is going, and acknowledges fear of falling. Mobility is also impaired by the wearing of slippers due to long toenails. The home environment appears to lack safety equipment (adequate lighting, stair railings, bathtub safety railings). Although conscious of loss of appetite, she appears unaware of weight loss despite wearing clothes that are too loose. Further testing failed to confirm memory loss but did indicate severe depression. Mrs. G. revealed some awareness of the motivational basis of her occupational dysfunctions by commenting positively about her skill during performance testing.

Mrs. G.'s activities have been based primarily in the home and immediate neighborhood. Social contacts have been reduced as a result of self-imposed and real activity limitations and a failure to replace friendships curtailed by disability, death and relocation. Paid help does yard care, home repairs, and housekeeping tasks. Mrs. M., the daughter-in-law, is the sole provider of other types of practical assistance. Psychological support is available from the 4 daughters who reside a considerable distance from their mother. Despite Mrs. G.'s dependency in feeling that her children should take care of her as she did for them, she prefers to remain independent in her own home, lest she exhibit favoritism in choosing a daughter to live with. Mrs. M., is willing to continue providing intermittent but not daily care. She is feeling stressed by coping with: a part-time job, caring for her own mother as well as her mother-in-law, widowhood, "long-distance" instructions from her sisters-in-law, and the sense that Mrs. G. is taking advantage of her.

In summary, there has been a progressive deterioration of Mrs. G.'s daily living habits over the past 3 years, precipitated by the illness and death of her husband, and subsequently by the sudden death of her 2 sons. Despite skill disuse and perceptions of incompetence, Mrs. G.'s skills remain essentially intact. Mrs. G.'s occupational dysfunctions appear to be primarily of a motivational origin, although performance in some areas is hindered by visual and mobility impairments. Overall, Mrs. G. retains the skills needed for independent living, however problems in transportation, safe mobility and task performance, and social stimulation need to be resolved.

REFERENCES

Beck, A.T., Ward, C.H., Mendelson, M., Mock, J., Erbaugh, J. (1961). An inventory for measuring depression. Archives of General Psychiatry, 4, 53–63.

Blazer, D. (1982). *Depression in late life.* St. Louis, MO: C.V. Mosby.

Csuka, M., McCarty, D.J. (1985). Simple method for measurement of lower extremity muscle strength. The American Journal of Medicine, 78, 77–81.

Folstein, M.F., Folstein, S., McHugh P.R. (1975). Mini-mental state: A practical method for grading the cognitive state of patients for the clinician. Journal of Psychiatric Research, 12, 189–198.

Hamilton, M. (1967). Development of a rating scale for primary depressive illness. British Journal of Social and Clinical Psychology, 6, 278–296.

Tinetti, M.E. (1986). Performance-oriented assessment of mobility problems in elderly patients. Journal of the American Geriatrics Society, 34, 119–126.

Verwoerdt, A. (1976). *Clinical geropsychiatry.* Baltimore, MD: The Williams & Wilkins Company.

Yesavage, J.A., Brink, T.L., Rose, T.L., Lum, O., Huan, V., Adey, M.B., Leirer, V.O. (1983). Development and validation of a geriatric depression rating scale: A preliminary report. Journal of Psychiatric Research, 17, 37–49.

Zung, W.W.K. (1965). A self-rating depression scale. Archives of General Psychiatry, 12, 63–70.

Mastery and Achievement: Guidelines Using Clinical Problem Solving With Depressed Elderly Clients

Helen Smith, Dip OT

> The continued psychological well being of the aged, similar to the needs of persons at all stages of life, is largely dependent upon a high level of activity, involvement with other persons and with interests beyond their own personal lives. (Sussman, 1976, as cited by Jackson, 1983)

INTRODUCTION

The theoretical framework for this paper is the model of human occupation which emphasizes the importance of people being involved in doing at all stages of life, from infancy through adulthood and on to the very end of life. The model of human occupation gives rise to an organizing paradigm which serves to foster understanding of the dynamics and the salience of human achievement to mental health in old age.

In examining mental health in aging, the concept of human stress will be introduced. The relationship between stress and depression, especially in the later years will be discussed.

Helen Smith is a lecturer in the School of Occupational Therapy, Cumberland College of Health Sciences, Sydney, N.S.W., Australia.

Based on a presentation made at the International Symposium: Occupational Therapy Approaches to Depression in Older Adults, Pre-Congress Conference, XIII International Congress of Gerontology, July, 1985, Columbia University, New York.

The author wishes to thank Dr. Richard Geeves for his willing support at all times and his permission to use the Hornsby-Ku-ring-gai Hospital NHLT as her case study. The author gratefully acknowledges the advice and encouragement received from Lesley Blackett, Mairi Grant, Ruth Beltran, Janet Bell and Tony Koop.

This paper draws together and synthesizes afresh current thinking about aging and in so doing it provides a rationale and guidelines for the organization of treatment and support systems for elderly individuals suffering from depression.

Aged care is addressed in the context of mastery versus helplessness. A pilot project involving specific treatment strategies and techniques is presented. This project offers a prototype for management of elderly clients organized around the use of services and support systems within the community.

HUMAN OCCUPATION AND ACTION

Human occupation has been described as "an innate, spontaneous tendency of the human system to explore and master the environment" (Kielhofner & Burke, 1980:573). The implication is that human beings throughout their life are involved in choosing and exploring environmental settings. The model of human occupation further postulates that individuals develop competence by involvement in these settings which allows them to perform an increasing number and range of occupational activities (Kielhofner & Burke, 1980).

According to Fidler (1978) all organisms are equipped to act, from the smallest, simplest form of life to the most complex. She points out that as human beings we are equipped with basic behavioral patterns which allow us to cope with the environment. However, in comparison with the simpler forms of life, humans are very dependent upon the social and cultural environments for learning. Fidler asserts that human action is necessary and essential for human existence and survival.

Current research on activity is addressing the relationship between neurological processes and motor behavior. Significant data is beginning to emerge which supports the concept that the drive for action, translated into an ability to do, is fundamental to ego development and adaptation (Fidler, 1978).

Activity or action is closely connected to the concept of human occupation. Action is behavior motivated by an intrinsic, conscious urge to be effective in the environment. This effectiveness is demonstrated in the performance of individually interpreted roles, shaped by cultural tradition, and learned through a process of socialization (Burke, 1983 as cited by Kielhofner, 1983b).

In occupational therapy, action is equated with doing. Doing is the process of experimenting and trying out. It is gaining experience by creating, controlling, choosing, managing, responding, performing, effecting, transacting and bringing about. It is through such action with feedback from the environment that a person comes to know the potentials and limitations of self and the surrounding world. Achieving competence in the environment and establishing feelings of intrinsic worth are dependent upon the process of doing (Fidler, 1978). Action is a lifelong and fluctuating process of doing and receiving feedback.

Rogers (Kielhofner, 1983b) proposes that a need and tendency to explore and master surrounding environments gives rise to the development of competence in performing an increasing number and range of activities. The assumption is that body and mind are interconnected, implying that *action* is necessary for maintenance of both mental and physical function and thus for health. This assumption is the basis on which occupation, i.e. action, is used as a therapeutic means to maintain health or to restore function.

The Aging Process

Aging is invariably accompanied by changes in physical function which can lead to lower levels of activity and decreased competence in performance. Such age related changes are relatively benign and characteristically have a gradual onset which permits adaptation to changing capacities. There are however pathological processes associated with age which tend to be chronic in nature and to manifest with significant loss of functional ability. When this occurs, maintaining an effective level of occupational behavior becomes a problem necessitating therapeutic intervention.

In addition to the loss of physical capacity, mild or profound, which accompanies aging there are social losses such as the death of a spouse which add significant stress to an already stressed individual. The aged individual may be forced to relocate which may trigger a reactive depression.

An individual, having to withdraw from their familiar community, sever support networks and retreat into alternative accommodations can suffer extreme loss. A change in living situation precipitates the loss of identity and role and this, coupled with the original precipitating factor, can create great stress. Other aged individuals may become isolated from the familiar environment by problems of mobility and frailty thus becoming virtual prisoners within their own homes. These crisis situations are becoming more and more frequent particularly among those over the age of 80 years.

Learned Helplessness and Depression

Seligman (1975) has developed a learned helplessness model of depression. He postulates that reactive depression can result from learned helplessness. This situation can occur when individuals have lost control over gratification and relief from suffering and believe themselves to be powerless and helpless. They see the future as bleak. When exposed to events beyond their control individuals learn that responding is futile. Consequently, incentives to respond are undermined, thus producing a lessening of motivation. The result of this conditioning can be mental disorders. Behaviorally the individual reacts with passivity, submission and depression (Seligman, 1975).

Approximately 68% of the elderly admitted to psychiatric services are suffering from depression. It is estimated that 14% of the elderly will suffer from a severe depression at some stage during their latter years (Jackson, 1983).

Psychodynamic Paradigm

Solomon and Goldfarb (Jackson, 1983) propose a treatment approach to counteract feelings of helplessness and dependency. They propose the activation of internalized feelings through the use of graded behavioral tasks which guarantee clients' success. This approach allows the individual to regain mastery and control over their environment. By ensuring that the clients make all the decisions about basic daily tasks, Soloman claims that clients will achieve and accept responsibility for the behaviors they display. Solomon asserts that continued access to and help from personal support systems of families and friends with the continued option of risk taking will contribute to the clients having a renewed sense of choice and control.

Solomon proposes that the elderly experience a variety of stresses which can trigger a characteristic sequence of coping events. These stresses can happen at any age but are more likely and usually more concentrated in the elderly. These stresses involve losses of various types such as loss of spouse, children and livelihood, loss of social role, health, mobility, income, and housing. Inadequate opportunities for leisure activities as well as lack of an alternative to work can cause a profound sense of loss in the aged individual.

The social victimization inflicted on the elderly by governmental policies on pensions and assets or by negative societal attitudes towards aging can also affect the elderly person adversely. Feelings of increased helplessness and dependence can be reinforced and compounded by health care workers, influenced perhaps, by negative stereotyping and aging concepts which can lead the client to adopt the "sick role." The power differential inherent in the interpersonal relationships between client and therapist can contribute to client dependency if used inappropriately and negatively.

Thus it is apparent that the elderly may experience a diminished sense of mastery over their environment and a loss of control over their destiny, with feelings of increased helplessness and ambivalent feelings of dependency.

INTERVENTION

The growing proportion of elderly in our population makes it increasingly imperative to respond to the health needs of aged clients. The goals for treatment of the elderly client may need to be reassessed. It may not be possible to restore the elderly individual to full independence. Different, limited goals of optimizing function to provide a greater degree of human dignity and happiness may be a more realistic objective for treatment. The provision of support services within a community form a necessary adjunct to treatment programs for the elderly and should be viewed as an adjunct to living which helps to maintain hard won mobility and independence (Ford, 1981, as cited by Howe, 1981).

Independent Living Rehabilitation for the Elderly

One effective way of rethinking and refocusing intervention for the elderly is through the use of Independent Living Rehabilitation Programs. Jackson and Lang (Jackson, 1983) describe Independent Living Rehabilitation (ILR) as having control over one's life based on the choice of acceptable options that minimize reliance on others in making decisions and in performing everyday activities. ILR promotes self-help consumer involvement and helps to prevent premature and inappropriate institutional care for the disabled elderly. The priorities of ILR are to promote an appropriate level of independence and community living.

Independence is a relative concept which may be defined and interpreted differently by each individual. In modern society an individual's ability to be self-sufficient is usually encouraged from childhood. Adults are supposed to have learned to depend upon themselves. Yet consider that few individuals live alone in the world. We are to a lesser or greater degree interdependent with others. We have times of need when we desire some relative degree of dependence. In practice, our concept and interpretation of functional and physical independence is as varied as individuals are one from another. By the same token we also need reasonable control over our own life, based on the choice of acceptable options that minimize reliance on others. Let us not deny this need to our aging clients!

The conflict between dependency and helplessness, and the rehabilitation goals that emphasize autonomy, independence and minimization of disability are very real and must be addressed by all health professionals when working with the elderly. Do we really desire full autonomy and complete mastery for our clients or would we prefer them to be somewhat dependent upon us and our care thus perpetuating our usefulness and satisfying our needs for self-fulfillment and self-esteem? This conflict of expectations must be clearly defined and recognized especially when working with the elderly. The sociocultural norms and expectations of aging and the aging process emphasize the dilemma of providing care versus fostering independence. The cost effectiveness of intervention, the use of scarce resources at a time of diminishing supply and increasing demands, all contribute to the growing dilemma of providing rehabilitation services to elderly individuals.

If we decide that mastery and choice are the goals for elder client care and if the resources available will sustain these goals, we must guard against perpetuating learned helplessness and depression. It is possible to enable clients to overcome the very real stresses they experience and facilitate independence in community living.

Community Living

The current philosophy of aged care in Australia is changing to a more community orientated focus away from institutional care. For our elderly clients the situation may offer many more options for care and support within their own homes in the community. As appealing as this idea is, it is not without hazard. For some elders such care could prove disastrous.

Home based, community care may well result in a population of frail aged, living alone and isolated from interaction with others by the barriers of access, transport and workforce limitations. This group of isolated, frail elderly people can very quickly become a population disengaged from society, resulting in helplessness and depression, unless appropriate, effective and sufficient support systems are organized and coordinated.

How can we assist elder clients to maintain their optimum dignity and integrity? How can we prevent helplessness occurring in two very different environments—the nursing home and the private home?

Several years ago, the Health Commission in Australia recognized the need for a clearly articulated philosohy of aged care at the institutional level as well as within the community. A pilot study was initiated in 1977 in the northern metropolitan areas of Sydney, N.S.W., Australia. The goal of the program was twofold: to assess the need for and to provide activity programs in nursing homes and to assess the need for a peer review system to be set up for nursing home staff.

PILOT PROGRAM

The Health Commission began the pilot study with the objective of: "ensuring residents of nursing homes live as normal a life as possible within the limits of their disabilities, with the resulting decreased dependence on staff" (Memo from Health Commission, 1977). Nursing homes in the northern metropolitan area of Sydney are primarily privately owned and run with registered nurses-in-charge. The majority of other staff are untrained nursing assistants. The opportunities for inservice programs and continuing education had previously been minimal. To remedy this situation, the Health Commission established teams of health care professionals to act as nursing home liaisons. The teams were responsible for establishing training programs whose goal was improvement of care giving and the quality of life for institutionalized and community living elders.

The Nursing Home Liaison Team (NHLT)

In the Hornsby Kuring-gai health region of N.S.W., Australia the NHLT team consisted of a nurse, an occupational therapist and an activity officer. The NHLT worked with three nursing homes who volunteered to participate in the pilot project in each area. The team assessed the specific needs within their area and identified their objectives as being:

1. To promote and provide resources and support systems for nursing home and hostel residents and staff.
2. To provide educational programs.
3. To enhance community awareness of aged person's care.

The NHLT had different roles in the nursing homes and in the community. Within nursing homes the team endeavored to:

1. assess the nursing home and advise on the use of community resources;
2. assess each resident and advise about appropriate assistive devices and transfer techniques;

3. educate staff in the utilization of and access to community and hospital based health resources;
4. advise on appropriate recreational activities for nursing home residents.

Within the community the NHLT team had involvement with:

1. Recruiting, interviewing, placing and supporting volunteers.
2. Training volunteers who worked in the community day activity clubs for the frail aged, chronically ill and handicapped.
3. Co-ordinating programs of dance and music for nursing home residents and activity club members.
4. Co-ordinating voluntary transport services for the elderly's health care appointments and activity program participation.

Education of health care providers, establishment of community support groups and participation in programs was an important focus of attention for the NHLT team working with patients, staff and volunteers in nursing homes and day center programs.

Evaluation of Pilot Program

Establishment of the NHLT resulted in improved co-ordination of aged services within the area, an increased community awareness of the needs of aged persons and an increased awareness and use of community resources.

At the end of six months, the pilot project evaluation demonstrated differences in behavior and attitude of both nursing home patients and staff. Fifty-six percent of elder patients showed improvement in their attitudes towards each other and the program and a 59 percent improvement was noted in elders' performance of activities of daily living skills.

Prior to the introduction of the NHLT thorough patient assessments were rarely completed in the nursing home. Nursing home staff themselves identified a lack of accurate assessment on admission, a situation which can perpetuate and increase dependence in patients. Residents' physical abilities have improved due to the work of the visiting therapist which has alleviated and improved existing problems.

Residents' emotional status and social interactions have also improved as a result of the NHLT activities. Patients, staff and visitors spontaneously commented that nursing home patients seem more at ease and happier with fewer quarrels and greater friendliness towards each other.

Following evaluation of the pilot project, the NHLT was implemented as an ongoing program. It has now been in operation for over eight years and the impact of the team has been considerable. They have been invited into many local nursing homes in the private sector where they have implemented patient assessments, activity programs, staff education programs and have provided support structures for staff.

The NHLT'S educational programs for activity officers from nursing homes have been regularly over-subscribed each year and have provided these caregivers with increased knowledge and skills of a variety of activities and processes. The elders' participation in activities has increased greatly at all levels—passive and active—and patients have topics to discuss and anticipation of future "happenings."

The presence of the NHLT within the homes is now welcome and this acceptance of the team and their goals has increased staff awareness of the residents' social needs as well as their nursing care needs. Staff have increased their sensitivity to the interrelationship between social and physical needs relative to the quality of life of residents.

In the community the NHLT's many educational programs have equipped volunteers and care takers to maintain community day centers and community outreach for the aged and disabled living in their own homes in the community. In this way elders in need within the community are sustained, thus avoiding the common pitfalls of isolated, dependent and depressed elderly in the community.

These findings emphasize the value and importance of the doing process and involvement for all aged persons, whether within the nursing home population or living in the community. It is the doing process which enables us all to gain mastery and achievement in our environment. Like all of us, the aged person has the need and right to be a useful, contributing member of a community for the whole of their life.

The importance of the liaison and coordination functions carried out by the NHLT has been vital in improving effective and efficient care. The teams have brought together relevant aged care services in the area. They have also educated the long term care personnel to improve the quality of aged care services. Now, many of our active aged in the community are successfully and competently involved in providing volunteer services. The functional elders provide valuable and essential services, giving them the opportunity to offer care and support to others.

SUMMARY AND CONCLUSIONS

As occupational therapists we are committed to the belief that people are active beings, whose development is influenced by the use of purposeful activity. Using the capacity for intrinsic motivation, therapists believe that humans are able to influence their physical environment through purposeful activity. Life involves a process of continuous adaptation and adaptation involves a change in function that promotes survival and self-actualization. Purposeful activity facilitates the adaptative response.

With our philosophic framework firmly based on occupation and with the focus of our concern on doing, the selection of the model of human occupation for this paper has special significance for treatment of the elderly client.

The therapist assesses the aged individual's needs and then establishes a context or environment in which the individual can experience mastery. A depressed elderly client with all the psychodynamics of learned helplessness, rolelessness, stress and loss can be given the opportunity of mastering this environment through choice and control options, and involvement in the process.

Negative social attitudes to aging are gradually changing. The aged themselves are more able, due to better education and increased numbers to stand up for themselves. Their political influence is stronger and they are better able to articulate their demands. Aged care is gradually losing its lower status position in the workforce.

Occupational therapists have a particular contribution to make in elder care. We can restore to our aging clients a faith in themselves, and can re-establish their sense of competence and mastery of their environment.

The importance of engagement and participation in life right to its end must be emphasized and encouraged. Occupation can be a means of restoring structure and time frames, meaning and role back into clients' lives. The model of human occupation can be used systematically to conceptualize clients' needs in all aged care services.

If we, as health workers, are genuinely concerned about our aging clients within our services, we must rethink our values and philosophies regarding aging and confront the very real issues of learned helplessness, dependence and depression.

Those practitioners with genuine concern for the elderly's quality of living, must focus on the needs of clients to obtain mastery and achievement in their daily lives and thus facilitate optimum mental health for each elderly person.

REFERENCES

Fidler, G. and Fidler, J. Doing and becoming. Purposeful action and self actualization. *American Journal of Occupational Therapy,* 1978, *32,* 305–310.

Health Commission of N.S.W. Memorandum, 1977. Sydney, Australia.

Howe, A. (ed.). *Towards an Older Australia.* 1981, Australia: University of Queensland Press.

Jackson, O. (ed.). *Physical Therapy of the Geriatric Patient.* 1983, U.S.A.: Churchill Livingstone, Inc.

Kielhofner, G. A heritage of activity: development of theory. *American Journal of Occupational Therapy,* 1983a, *36,* 723–729.

Kielhofner, G. *Health through occupation: Theory and practice in occupational therapy.* 1983b, U.S.A.: F.A. Davis Co.

Kielhofner, G. and Burke, J. A model of human occupation. Part I. Conceptual framework and content. *American Journal of Occupational Therapy,* 1980, *34,* 572–581.

Russell, C. *The ageing experience.* 1981, Sydney: George Allen & Unwin Aus. Pty. Ltd.

Seligman, M. *Helplessness. On depression, development and death.* 1975, U.S.A.: Freeman & Co.

Shaw, M. (ed.). *The challenge of ageing.* 1984, Melbourne: Churchill Livingstone.

Solomon, K. and Goldfarb, A. Psychosocial dysfunction in the aged. Cited in Jackson, O. (ed.). *Physical therapy of the geriatric patient.* 1983, U.S.A.: Churchill Livingstone.

An Expanded Community Role for Occupational Therapy: Preventing Depression

Alisa Ofsevit Eilenberg, MS, OTR

INTRODUCTION

Depression is a formidable illness currently threatening the well-being of countless community elderly. Their social isolation, the physical changes of aging and a societal focus on youth and the roles and skills of the young cause this group to be particularly vulnerable to depression. Therapeutic approaches employed by occupational therapists can be effectively applied to promote mental health and prevent depression in the community elderly.

After several years of working with institutionalized elderly psychiatric patients, many of whom had been admitted for depression, the author's focus turned to prevention stimulated by a course taken in the advanced Occupational Therapy Program at Columbia University.* As part of a related practicum at a senior center, the author designed and implemented a time-limited program to foster independence and prevent depression, as well as to observe the multidisciplinary efforts being made toward this end on an experimental basis. This preparation helped in the planning of the theoretical and practical aspects of the "Wellness Program" now carried out at the Mamaroneck Senior Center in Westchester.

Based on a presentation made at the International Symposium: Occupational Therapy Approaches to Depression in Older Adults, Pre-Congress Conference, XIII International Congress of Gerontology, July, 1985, Columbia University, New York.

* "Life Skills Reinforcement and its Relationship to Independent Living for the Elderly," Patricia Miller, MEd, OTR, 1984.

FRAMES OF REFERENCE

The "Wellness Program" is based on several frames of reference that form a comprehensive approach to preventing depression and promoting the health of the community elderly. The first frame of reference is developmental. Erikson, as cited in Belkin, described the chief challenge of old age as a struggle of "ego identity versus despair." Successful resolution of this life stage involves a sense of peace and acceptance of life's accomplishments and failures, an overall sense that one's life has been worthwhile. He suggests that depression results if this perspective is not attained (1980). Peck, as cited in Weiner, elaborates on Erikson's view by listing more specific tasks of old age, including adaptation to work and family role changes by the establishment of varied, valued activities. He stresses the importance of transcending physical and cognitive limitations and discomforts while enjoying social interaction. A further task is the focusing on making some contribution to the welfare of future generations rather than the preoccupation with death that so often accompanies depression (1978). The Wellness Program seeks to help members attain these goals and overcome the limitations of aging as each individual finds him or herself at a different point of development.

A sensory-integrative frame of reference focuses on the human need for adequate, varied and meaningful stimulation. Ideally, this input is then processed by the brain and permits daily adaptive behavior. Sensory integration is typically compromised in the elderly. Sensory systems such as sight, hearing, taste and smell are commonly diminished. The sense of joint movement and position in space may be impaired because of arthritic changes and reduced nerve conduction. The consequences of these changes are frequently slowed and cautious movement and decreased overall activity.

Socialization, a most important type of sensory and mental stimulation, is also compromised in the aged. This is due to death and relocation of friends, relatives (particularly spouses) and the scarcity of extended family systems in this society.

The author's previous research into the sensory-integrative needs of the elderly indicates that disuse of existing sensory-motor abilities only accelerates the deterioration of these systems. The inactivity and withdrawal that can accompany these losses puts the elderly at great risk of depression. Numerous studies of sensory deprivation demonstrate that inadequate stimulation and/or processing of information have devastating physical, cognitive and emotional effects, including vulnerability to disease, confusion, decreased motor skills, irritability and general withdrawal (Ofsevit, 1980).

Given the importance of sensory-integrative function, it is crucial that these needs be addressed in any program designed to prevent depression in the elderly. In the Wellness Program, a dance and movement part of each session is an important tool in meeting sensory-integrative needs of members.

A learning model is another useful frame of reference in the design of the Wellness Program. There is an assumption that given the motivation new skills can be learned and changes made in a lifestyle late in life. Mosey (1971) states that learning takes place as a consequence of positive reinforcement. In the Wellness Group, the reinforcement includes peer and leadership support for constructive changes, as well as the innate satisfaction that comes from mastery of one's environment. The forming of individualized goals, which, when met, increase members' sense of their autonomy, is a valuable approach to preventing the sense of helplessness that so often accompanies depression. The group problem-solving approach is a useful means to this end.

An additional frame of reference is the systems approach. This approach is useful in understanding the structure of any organization: staffing patterns, membership composition, goals, mandates, constraints of the institution. It was helpful in initially determining how occupational therapy skills could be applied toward furthering the existing goals of the senior center through the implementation of a new program and in maintaining open lines of communication for the ongoing success of the program.

PROGRAM SETTING

The Mamaroneck Senior Center has a membership of approximately two hundred from the Westchester area. It provides hot lunches Monday through Friday, daily activities, special events, and referrals for members in need of community services. Mamaroneck Human Resources is particularly involved in this regard. Staffing includes a chief administrator, site manager, a secretary, assistants, kitchen workers, as well as volunteers and consultants who conduct activity programs. The senior center is supported by federal funds which are scheduled to be gradually phased out, as well as by the town of Mamaroneck. Local community organizations frequently contribute toward special needs or events at the center.

The senior center aims to meet the social and recreational needs of its membership. There is also an awareness of the increasing frailty of members and the difficulties faced by them in terms of remaining well and independent in the community. The administrators were thus receptive to the idea of a Wellness Program which would have the aim of promoting health in this group at risk for physical deterioration, social isolation, and depression.

In introducing the Wellness Program at the center the author described the role of occupational therapists in different settings and with varied age groups. Life tasks change with the aging process. Older adults have tremendous adjustments to make to role changes, as children leave home, retirement arrives, and a spouse dies. The many physical changes that occur with aging often begin to interfere with the performance of daily activities. The purpose of the Wellness Program was to help older people make the fullest possible use of their abilities and to stay well and able to live in the community as long as possible.

An open discussion and written survey were provided to determine the unique health concerns of this population. Large and small group meetings were held as well as two consecutive sessions with individuals. Physical concerns expressed included arthritis, managing household tasks, improving posture, coping with pain, and getting adequate exercise. Psychosocial subjects of concern included living alone, using time more fully, and meeting new friends.

Following the written survey, members were invited to sign up for the Wellness Group. Potential participants were encouraged to give the group a try. The group was to be conducted in time-limited phases, after which members were free to continue or to leave. Individuals were pleased to know that the program would be geared to their needs, that no one would be pressured to participate beyond what was comfortable for them. Staff was helpful in identifying individuals who could benefit from the program. The response was enthusiastic. So many members signed up that a waiting list had to be started.

METHODOLOGY

The Wellness Group's objectives were influenced by the expressed needs of the population. This approach fostered the objectives of helping participants to discover and make use of their strengths, express their health needs and thus to realize the impact they can have on shaping their lives and environment. Another objective is for group members to form a supportive network of friendships at the senior center. A further objective is for members to gain and share knowledge about preserving physical abilities and compensating for deficits as these relate to activities of daily living. Yet another objective is for participants to understand a balanced, fulfilling use of time for them personally.

The group has a maximum enrollment of fifteen members per eight-week phase; each phase covers a specific topic. Every group begins with a one-hour discussion, using a group problem-solving approach. A half-hour of movement follows, including posture, breathing and warmup exercises along with selected ballroom, folk and free style expressive dance. The author meets with individuals during the final half hour. At the end of each eight-week phase, members are asked to assess the program via discussion and written survey.

The senior center's site manager helps publicize the group through the monthly calendar, weekly announcements and an attitude of enthusiastic support. Senior center staff set up the group's meeting area in advance. Periodic meetings are held with the site manager and the chief administrator to discuss the outcome of the group, and any difficulties or questions that arise.

The Wellness Group meets in the one long, large, often crowded room that comprises the temporary accommodations for the senior center during its renovation. A corner of the room is set up with a record player and a circle of chairs. Tables are pushed away to allow for needed space. The membership is asked to assist the group by keeping their voices lower than usual, since a high noise level interferes with discussion.

SAMPLE SESSIONS

Physical discomforts and increasing dependency that stem from arthritic conditions so common in the elderly can produce feelings of depression. The first series of sessions was devoted to arthritis and learning joint protection concepts, since this was the main priority indicated in the initial survey. Topics covered included resources for relieving and coping with pain, safety and management issues around the home, posture and body mechanics, and resources for coping with arthritis.

The theme of one particular session was finding a balance between rest and activity. The group was asked how they determined whether a household or other task was too much for them to handle. One woman described the enormous task of cleaning her fish tank. She had made it more manageable by emptying it out cup by cup. It was still exhausting and she felt that the only solution was to give up having the fish. Although this solution would be acceptable if the fish were no longer important to her, it was suggested that an alternative might be found if an effort were made to creatively solve the problem. That led to the topic of when, whom and how to ask for help. Possible resources, such as family and friends, were mentioned. The group discussed the advantages of calling upon them, the "price paid" for doing so or for not doing so. The importance of the timing of a request was discussed, along with consideration of the resource person's mood and obligations.

The tone of voice and attitude of the person making the request were explored. Participants pointed out that a demanding or hurried tone could make others less willing to help. It was also noted that firm self-advocacy was at times needed in case of hazards, such as when one member's window would not close during a harsh winter.

Mamaroneck Human Resources was mentioned as an additional resource. Members had heard that high school students and retirees were available for assistance with heavy tasks such as household repairs and that senior center staff might know more about specifics.

The group concluded with posture, breathing, and warmup exercises. There was dancing in pairs and as a group to oldtime jazz. All were encouraged to take part within their individual limitations and capacities. The mood of the group was lighthearted and cheerful. There was much enthusiastic participation.

The second phase of the Wellness Program dealt with developmental social concerns that can be handled constructively or make the elderly more vulnerable to depression. In this sample session, the group discussed the benefits and drawbacks of living alone. One member said that she thought it was fine for younger people to live alone, but that she would not want to do so at this time of life. Another woman had managed to live alone with no difficulty for many years. After her marriage late in life, however, when her husband was hospitalized, she found it a shock and nerve-wracking to suddenly be alone again.

One participant is usually withdrawn, in pain and has memory problems. He complained that it was terrible to live alone. When the group suggested he consider taking in a "boarder," he was emphatic that such a step would impinge on his freedom and independence. He didn't want to answer to anyone or be dictated by their needs. The group laughed in response to his description of some of the benefits of living alone.

A member whose husband lives in an institutional setting expressed her contentment with the flexibility of living alone. No one tells her when to go to sleep or get up, and she feels able to find all the company she needs outside of her home. Her one concern was security. She had worked to improve the building's security by fighting to get a front entrance lock, and so was no longer afraid of break-ins.

The group discussed security problems and measures to be taken, including getting a free security appraisal by the police.

Another member of the group had never married. Living alone was never a problem until recently, when she began to feel the need to have "someone around." We discussed the fact that needs often change over time. The group discussed housing alternatives and the fact that many older people are trying group living situations and taking in roommates.

The movement session following the discussion included warmups, dancing in pairs to square dance music, and free-style expressive dance.

Other topics covered in this phase were members' work and family backgrounds, current living situations, relocating, and making friends later in life.

Additional Group Topics

The extensive leisure time that older people are often faced with after retirement can be a source of new enjoyment or it can be a source of burdensome loneliness. A fulfilling use of time is quite important in preventing depression. It is vital in meeting sensory-integrative needs for variety and meaningful stimulation. A twelve-week phase of the program was devoted to the developmental task of exploring options to enhance or improve the use of time.

This particular session focused on adult education. The group was asked whether it was harder to learn earlier or later in life. One woman said she was concerned that she would not retain as much information now as she could when she was younger. Others had the same concern. We talked about ways to compensate for slight memory losses that affect many older people. One method mentioned was to have the instructor review material to reinforce learning. Other approaches discussed were practicing skills at home, reviewing with a classmate, and taking notes. It was pointed out that some types of courses such as film or music appreciation do not rely heavily on memory. It was noted that another aspect of successful learning later in life is one's attitude. If older students take a realistic and tolerant view of their abilities, they may enjoy the experience of learning without constantly comparing themselves to other learners.

Transportation as an issue that can help or interfere with taking classes was discussed. Accessibility and cost of transportation were considered. We discussed car pools, taxi pools, buses, and the possibility of exploring town funding to help older people attend classes.

The group concluded with exercise and dance to international folk music. Increased participation of members who had been reluctant to take part earlier was noted.

Additional topics covered during this phase were volunteer and work options, museums, theater and concert attendance, and other recreational options.

OBSTACLES ENCOUNTERED

Several factors have interfered with the group. One has been the physical setting of the Wellness Program. Leading a small group within a single, large and busy room has caused frequent distractions and interruptions. It poses a particular challenge to participants who are hearing impaired or distractible. This difficulty should be resolved with the completed renovation of the original senior center which will include small meeting rooms.

Another problem has been the varied demands on participants' schedules. In the community, events such as holiday preparation or even clothing sales can reduce attendance. Weather and illness inevitably interfere as well. Although flexibility is needed, participants should be reminded that attendance is a commitment and that each member is an important and valuable part of the group. The site manager has been most helpful in reinforcing the importance of attendance and in locating members who fail to attend.

Funding has severely limited the time that can be devoted to the Wellness Program. A more extensive program could reach more people, allow for more teaching and reinforcement of the kinds of adaptive skills mentioned earlier, and permit leadership in time-consuming projects that would benefit a large portion of the senior center membership.

ASSESSMENT OF THE PROGRAM

After the first eight-week phase of the group, a written survey was provided to assess the effectiveness of the group. Eleven of the thirteen regular members completed the survey. The following quotations are some representative responses to the questions, "How did the group benefit you, if at all?" and "Has the group influenced your lifestyle in any way?"

1. "I realized not to feel bad when I can't do ordinary things but to accept it and work around it. There always is a way." "I exercise more often."
2. "It helped to talk about the problem and bring it out in the open." "I realized I've got to get a little more exercise."
3. "It was a time to participate in the different exercises and to get to know the other people." "Made more friends, made me aware of how to help myself in many tasks, and to know where to look for help should I ever need it."

When asked how the group might be improved, participants who responded in the earlier survey expressed complete contentment with the structure of the group, praising the leadership as being motivating and enthusiastic. Only in the most recent survey were members at all critical. There were requests for a larger group, for craft instruction, and for more time to be devoted to movement. This suggests that over time, group members have become more secure and autonomous in terms of voicing their needs.

The group and leader have made various observations about members during the course of the sessions. The group spontaneously told one member who had been initially lethargic that she looked more awake and happy. Another participant reported feeling much more energetic after practicing some of the exercises at home. In time, this same group member took on greater responsibility within the senior center and demonstrated considerable creative abilities in that setting for the first time. Another participant who had always considered herself "just a listener" found that to her satisfaction, she was eventually able to express her own opinions. Two members began volunteer jobs in the course of the sessions, and one decided to take driving lessons in order to take fuller advantage of leisure options.

These changes occurred over weeks and months. The size and supportive nature of the group, as well as the structure, which is carefully tailored to address the needs of a specific group of older adults, has greatly helped members to make the most of their abilities and promote their health on many levels. Those who entered the group withdrawn and isolated clearly benefited from the program at least for short periods of time. Members who came with greater personal strengths have made fuller use of their resources and inspired their peers in the process.

IMPLICATIONS FOR OCCUPATIONAL THERAPY PRACTICE

There is a vast and increasing population of community elderly in need of preventive services. Some are obviously depressed, while many experience low levels of depression which are not dramatic, but nevertheless take a heavy toll in terms of socialization, disuse of existing living skills and physical abilities. Their potential contribution to their own welfare, to their families and communities is being lost.

Occupational therapists have the potential skill for organizing preventive programs. Our wholistic training provides a perspective on the developmental needs of each age group. Our schooling in the basic sciences gives us a grasp of the physical changes and sensory-integrative needs of old age. We are creative teachers equipped to assess individual needs, teach living skills, and motivate clients in the face of many obstacles.

Occupational therapy educational programs need to focus more on prevention and the burgeoning needs of the elderly. Training must include an understanding of and practical experience in community organizations to help therapists feel secure in noninstitutional settings.

At the highest levels of the professional association, occupational therapists must take an active role in paving the way for community practice. Most community organizations that serve the elderly either are unfamiliar with occupational therapy or associate any kind of therapy with hospitals and the ill. The scarcity of funds for new programs within community organizations makes it equally difficult if not impossible for occupational therapists to support themselves doing preventive work in the community.

As a professional body, occupational therapists need to lobby government officials and endeavor to educate the public about the at-risk community elderly and how our services might be used to keep older people independent and well in the community as long as possible.

Occupational therapy can and should assume a substantial role in preventive services for the elderly. Prevention programs address a relatively neglected area: keeping older people healthy. The possibility of preventing unnecessary use of more costly care needs to be carefully explored through research. The author's experience indicates that much of the isolation, despair, boredom, and physical deterioration that face the community elderly can be reduced and to some extent reversed by preventive occupational therapy programs.

REFERENCES

Belkin, Gary S., *An Introduction to Counseling*. (Dubuque, Iowa: Wm. C. Brown Company, 1980), pp. 262–263, 270, 280–281.

Mosey, Anne Cronin, *Three Frames of Reference for Mental Health*. 3rd ed. (Thorofare, New Jersey: Charles B. Slack, 1971), p. 109.

Ofsevit, Alisa, "The Effect of a Sensory Integration Movement Group on Life Satisfaction for the Frail Elderly (unpublished Occupational Therapy Master's Thesis, Columbia University, 1980).

Weiner, Marcella Bakur, Brok, Albert J., and Snadowsky, Alvin M., *Working with the Aged—Practical Approaches in the Institution and Community*. (Englewood Cliffs, New Jersey: Prentice-Hall, Inc., 1978), pp. 27–29.

BIBLIOGRAPHY

Burnside, Irene: *Working with the Elderly—Group Process and Techniques*. 2nd ed. Monterey, California: Wadsworth, Inc., 1984.

Butler, Robert and Lewis, Myrna: *Aging in Mental Health: Positive* Psychosocial *Approaches*. 3rd ed. St. Louis: C.V. Mosby Co., 1977.

Caplow-Lindner, Erna, Harpaz, Leah, and Samberg, Sonya: *Therapeutic Dance/ Movement—Expressive Activities for Older Adults*. New York: Human Sciences Press, 1979.

Steps in the Progressive Treatment of Depression in the Elderly

Fiona Docherty, Dip, COT

> Depression, depression, it follows my life it eats through my mind with its fears and its strife, it kills all the joy—forbidding all good reduces our work to no trees for the wood. My sleep is a fortune, a dread of the night, the need for oblivion just blocks out all light, a tiredness, proportions too great to relate is how one is ripped in this pendulous fate. I feel for all people who suffer as I, is the alternative to curl up and die?
>
> *Author Unknown*

INTRODUCTION

Depression in the elderly is often not acknowledged until the illness is well established. The general practitioner is the first link in the treatment chain. Referral is then made to the psychogeriatrician who assesses the patient at home before deciding on a course of action. If the depression is severe referral to the hospital is arranged. Patients expressing suicidal thoughts and having severe retardation of thinking and physical processes often require in-patient admission. If possible, the patient is referred to the Psychogeriatric Day Hospital for assessment and treatment. This allows the rehabilitation process to

---

Fiona Docherty, Royal Victoria Hospital, Edinburgh, Scotland.

Based on a presentation made at the International Symposium: Occupational Therapy Approaches to Depression in Older Adults, Pre-Congress Conference, XIII International Congress of Gerontology, July, 1985, Columbia University, New York.

start quickly, as the patient is not yet relinquishing responsibility and independence. Attendance is based on need; one to three days a week is the usual requirement, but this can be adjusted accordingly.

If the depression is mild and purely a socio-environmental reaction it may be more appropriate for referral to a local day centre, or club, for purely social contact. The day hospital, in contrast, provides the expertise of each discipline which the day centre cannot provide.

Occupational therapy is an integral part of the day hospital. The principles of occupational therapy in gerontology were in use in the early civilizations. Quality of life was stressed by Seneca in 3 B.C., who stated that life, rather than years, was important. Cicero in 43 B.C. presented a positive attitude towards ageing, recommending physical exercise, diet, and intellectual activities. All these requirements and more are being fulfilled today in the treatment of depression within the day hospital setting.

Day hospitals, first developed in Great Britain in 1946, have been increasing rapidly and add a worthwhile dimension to improving the quality of life of the elderly.

APPROACH TO TREATMENT

Every person is unique. Symptoms may be the same as those of fellow sufferers but no one has the same genes, upbringing and life experiences. Bearing this in mind, each patient is treated as an individual on a one to one or group basis, using the problem oriented approach. This approach takes a holistic view of the patient in relation to his psychological, physical, and socio-environmental needs, using the combined skills of the multidisciplinary team communicating and practising their particular expertise in assessment and treatment. Overlap inevitably occurs but this allows the possibility of sharing and receiving support from other team members. A cheerful, friendly, caring team gives an aura of success and confidence which projects onto the patients.

Problems, once identified, classified and given a priority rating are discussed at a weekly team meeting where treatment plans are formulated and other modes of treatment re-evaluated. The progression of care involves the following: home visits, activities of daily living, individual and group treatment, which includes outings to the community. The formation of community link groups is a vital step in the rehabilitation process (see Figure 1).

Home Visiting: The First Step

Home visiting plays an increasingly important part in the role of the occupational therapist in treating depression. Patients are assessed and constantly re-evaluated. It is more realistic to carry out this assessment in the patient's own familiar surroundings, allowing a treatment programme to be identified and started during the first home visit. The first step in treatment is the building up of rapport and trust

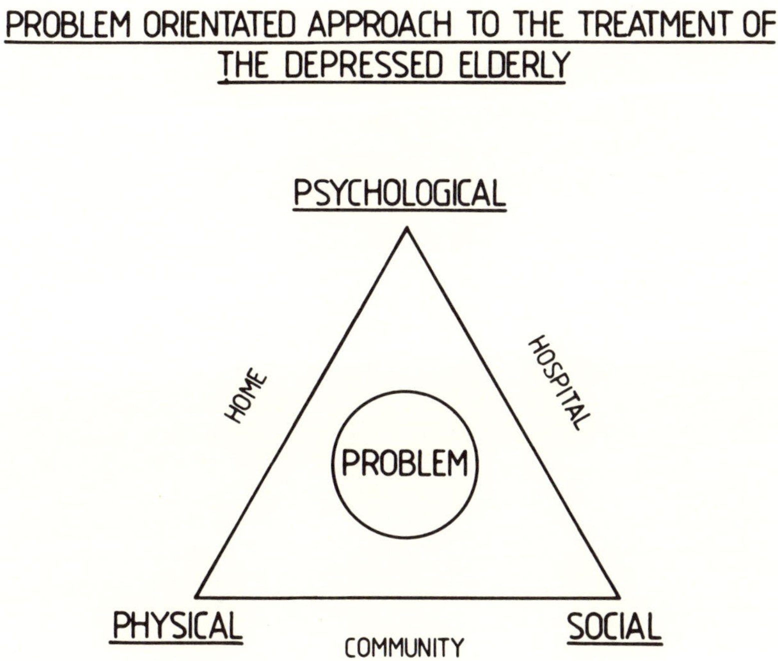

FIGURE 1

which is paramount and the basis of any realistic treatment programme.

Feelings of unworthiness and fear, the accompaniments of depression, respond well to replacing despair with hope and giving practical support. Initial introduction to the day hospital may sometimes be accomplished by first gaining the patient's confidence, explaining the function of the day hospital and by bringing the patient in the therapist's car for his/her first visit.

Home visiting can be divided into three types: the initial home visit; a follow-up visit allowing further assessment of the patient's functional ability, as well as encouragement to resume daily living activities. Finally, the routine unannounced visit which is extremely valuable, both as a support and re-assessment measure. It's amazing what you find when a patient least expects a visit. Working with relatives, supporters, home aides, friends and neighbors is of great value and helps bring about more lasting results.

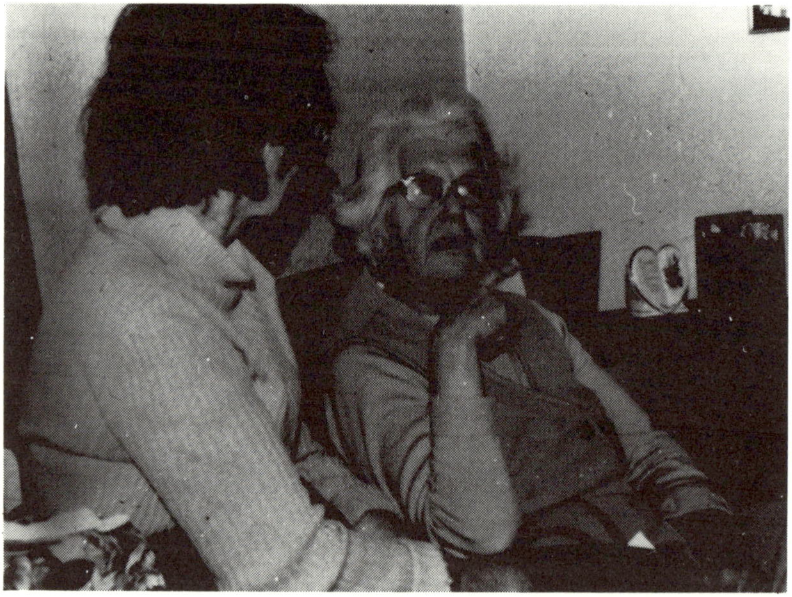

Attending to Individual Needs

Activities of Daily Living

Individual problems, e.g., inadequate diet caused by lack of motivation to shop and cook are tackled by the accomplishment of a simple meal within the hospital Activities of Daily Living suite. As the therapist's support is gradually withdrawn, and confidence is gained, some fellow patients might be invited to have a lunch shopped, cooked, and served by the patient. Confidence is thereby built up and relationships strengthened with positive reinforcement from all. Practise achieved in the supportive hospital setting can then be carried out at home.

Treatment Modules

Individual Treatment

The first part of a patient's treatment is involvement in the day hospital daily programme of intellectual, sensory and social stimulation, carried out by occupational therapy and nursing staff. All patients take part in this, first by being passively involved, later by becoming actively involved as they gain confidence. Exercises to music, quizzes, word games, seasonal entertainments and birthday celebrations form part of this general programme. Along with this, specific treatments are carried out by more senior team members of each discipline, either on an individual or a group basis. In addition to their psychological needs, physical problems relating to self care, sensory deficits, mobility, and other problems are referred to the appropriate department. The elderly have problems that are age related as well as a result of depression. Their special needs can best be met by having a wide variety of treatment modules available.

Communication among staff members, physician, family and community services is of vital importance and is the essence of cohesion and unity. It is an amalgam of all input that brings about lasting recovery.

Group Treatment

Group work plays a prominent part in treatment, and is carried out in separate rooms adjacent to the main day hospital area. Group work with the elderly has to be more structured, taking into consideration the reduction in their ability to handle abstract information. Older persons also find it harder to remember the meaning of what is being said as their information processing becomes slower.

The facility for recall is important as they have considerable life experiences behind them. Through participation in the groups, recall is stimulated and provides a basis for developing friendships and encouraging social interaction. Hearing and eyesight problems in addition require sensitivity in their positioning within the group. Groups are either psychotherapeutic groups that use no external media, for example, the feelings group, where free floating discussion takes place, or those using external media as in art, music and poetry groups, using projective techniques. Psycho-drama is also used at a later stage (see Figure 2).

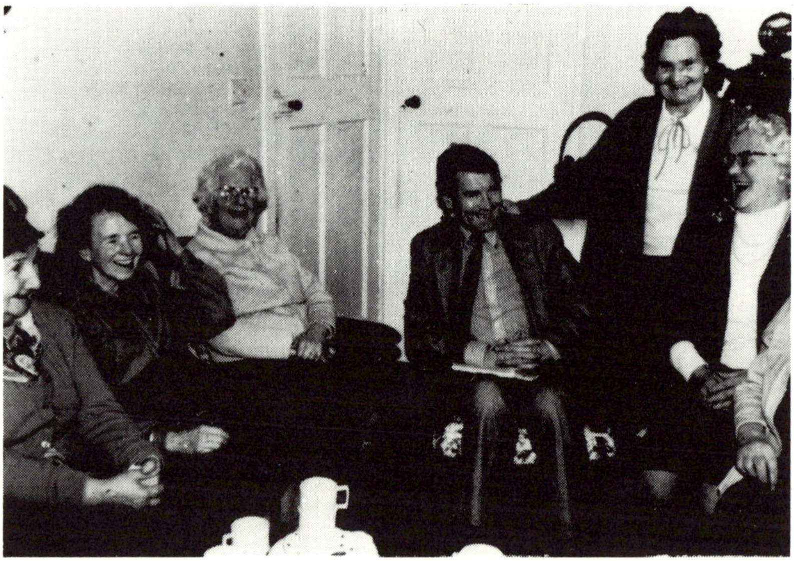

Group Spirit Prevails

TREATMENT:

GROUPS WITH THE ELDERLY

AIMS
1. LIBERATE AND EXPLORE FEELING
2. PROMOTE INSIGHT
3. ISOLATE PROBLEMS
4. MODIFY BEHAVIOUR
5. SET TARGETS
6. IMPROVE COMMUNICATION
7. PROMOTE CONFIDENCE
8. PROMOTE ADAPTABILITY
9. INITIATE SELF HELP CONCEPT
10. FOSTER CARING AND SHARING

FIGURE 2

THE AIMS of group work with the depressed elderly are to:

1. Liberate and explore feelings—hence the name FEELINGS GROUP;
2. Overcome inhibitions enabling repressed material to gain expression;
3. Promote insight without which there can be no change;
4. Modify behaviour;
5. Set targets and achieve goals;
6. Promote self confidence;
7. Promote adaptability to facilitate change;
8. Initiate a self help concept;
9. Foster caring and sharing;
10. Encourage socialisation.

Outings

Outings play a very valuable part in the assessment and rehabilitation of patients with a depressive illness, often sup-

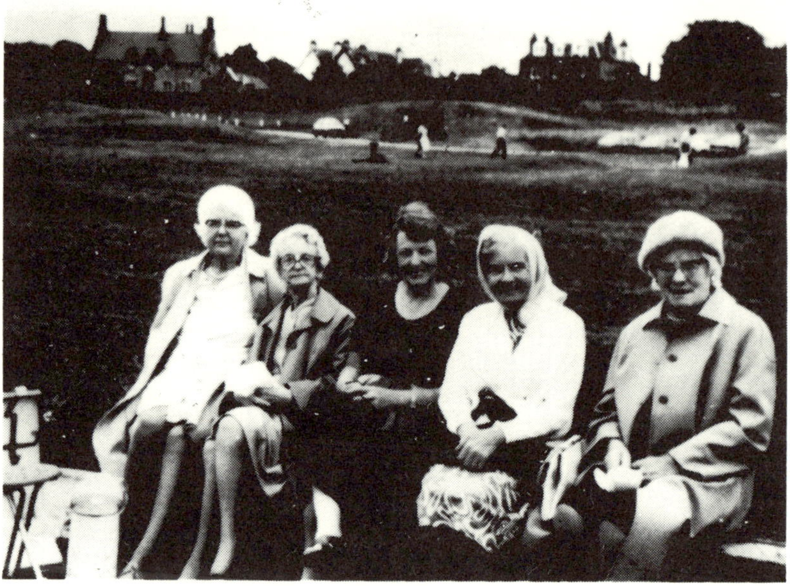

An Outing

plying the first necessary stimulation and motivation to lift their mood and give them an aim in life once more. Transport can be by hospital bus for a large group outing, or by therapist's car for an individual or small group outing. Outings can be divided into two main types. Purely *social outings* are of value in the initial stages of depression, providing a feeling of normality and enabling the therapist to build trust. They also provide further knowledge of the patient observed in the course of normal social interaction.

The second type of outing is *therapeutic* in concept, used later in the treatment in conjunction and as an extension of the psychotherapeutic group involvement. Individual problems can be worked through with practise given in a normal setting thus increasing the patients' self confidence. A trip to the local airport provides an excellent venue for tackling problems such as fear of using public transport, coping with crowds, using escalator and lift (elevator). Many elderly are frightened and need instructions to learn to operate the door hold mechanism. Feelings can be talked through and confidence gained.

Handling money and decision making can be practised by using self service facilities when ordering coffee and cake. The elderly can become housebound by being unable to overcome their anxieties and fears. Outings can provide the means to open the door to an improved quality of life and form a valuable therapeutic tool.

Problems can also be addressed on an individual basis. Lack of interest and motivation with accompanying anxiety, as well as lack of confidence and low self esteem, can best be tackled by building up a profile of the patient's life style in co-operation with his close associates and finding an activity that the patient used to enjoy. Treatment has to be graded, built up gradually, with constant re-evaluation. For example, a patient called Mary was taken on three successive visits to the local swimming pool. This was a progressive reintroduction of swimming, which was her previous interest before the onset of her depressive illness. This interest was a shared one with her husband. He was rapidly losing patience with her, and the author used this both as a means of building up her confidence, and of improving their relationship. Although her anxiety level was extremely high, she used to love swimming, so her motivation was good.

On the first occasion Mary was just able to sit on the steps of the swimming pool encouraged by a student therapist and the author. On the second occasion the therapists supported her while she timidly entered the water. Her confidence was growing slowly. On the third occasion she was able to walk across the shallow end. On the fourth occasion she swam. The delight on her face and the promotion of her self confidence was a joy to behold. Her husband was delighted, and replaced negative attitudes with positive ones, thus improving her confidence further.

Group psychotherapy has come to be regarded as one of the most important methods of treating patients with emotionally determined symptoms, abnormal behaviour and personality disorders. It is particularly effective in the treatment of depression. Its current position as an effective treatment is based on the contention that changes are more enduring with

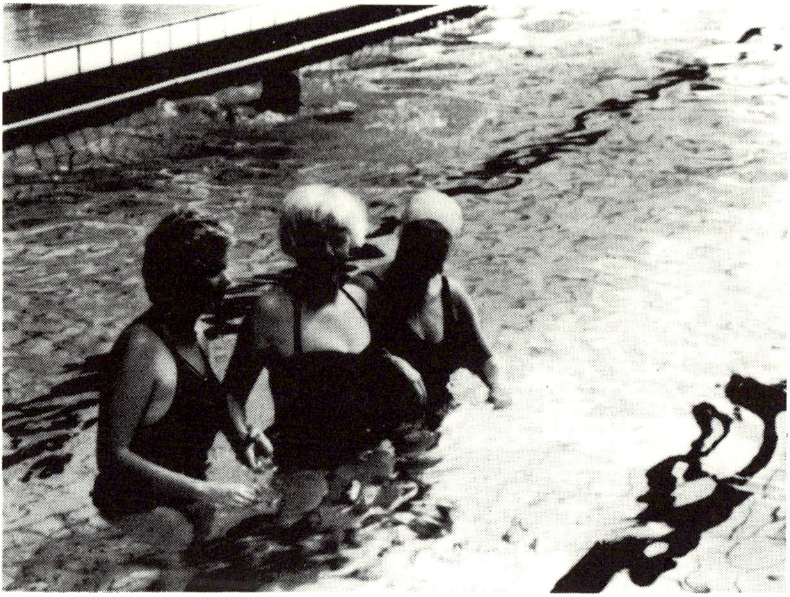

Returning to Familiar Pastimes

people treated in groups because their social relationships have improved.

Music Group

Music is a universal language and a social record of our times. Being the least threatening medium it can be used as an introduction to the psychotherapeutic group situation. It has a cathartic effect, freeing suppressed emotions and giving relief. Used in conjunction with verbal imagery it can be utilized to reduce tension, aid relaxation and relieve anxiety which so often is an accompaniment of depression. Memories have been found to be stored with their associated feelings; this being so, music triggering memories allows emotional release. Music has a spiritual quality with the power to uplift and inspire, thus helping to lift the mood of the severely depressed patients and satisfying their inner needs.

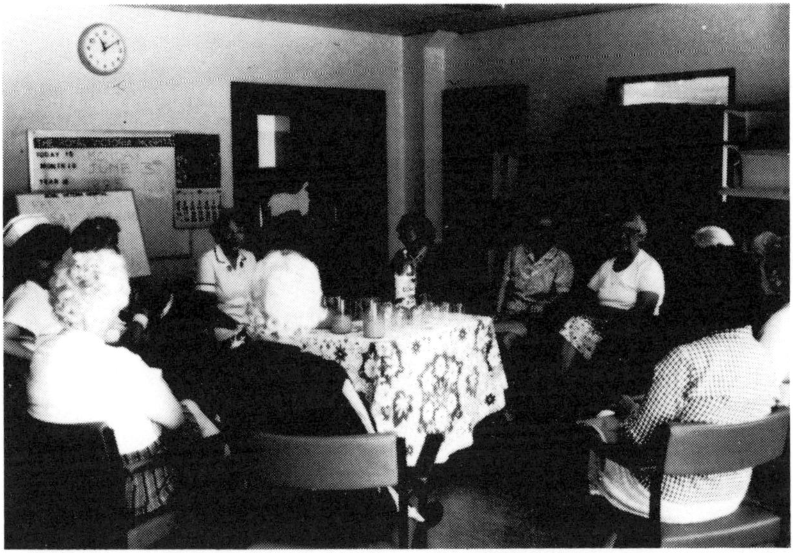

The Group Gathers for Coffee

Poetry

The Greeks recognized the healing power of poetry by having Apollo as the dual God of poetry and medicine. Poetry is the purest form of language and has been an instrument by which especially sensitive individuals in all lands and ages record their emotional upheaval and imaginative wanderings. Poetry may create order where chaos has existed, whether the chaos is in the patient himself or in his relationship with others. As a treatment medium its aim is to seek the meaning that the poem has for each individual patient, helping him reach levels of emotional insight more adequately than conventional dialogue. It facilitates catharsis in an accepting atmosphere, and provides an avenue for behaviour modification, especially in interpersonal relationships. An illustration of this is a poem, used when Annie, having quarrelled with all her friends, was very lonely and had no insight into her behaviour:

"THE QUARREL"

They haven't spoken for a week,
Both feel as much annoyed
—a week of life and love thus spoiled
that could have been enjoyed.
Both of them unhappy
Yet neither calls a truce,
but pride as a companion is of very little use.
Life is too short and love too rare to waste
a single day.
What does it matter who's to blame
So long as one give way.

A variety of poems can be used to arouse different emotions. Achieving a balance using humorous as well as serious poems can create a positive group feeling. Its value is that it presents a tangible structure allowing the patient to express his point of view without realising he is doing so, while also interpreting the poem. As such, it is an extremely suitable medium for group work with the depressed elderly who are resistant to talking about their own problems.

Art

Art can be used in several ways. First, as a medium in the psychotherapeutic groups using projective techniques where feelings can be explored and information about patients gained. Art is a much more threatening medium than either music or poetry and often has to be more structured, e.g., by dividing a page into two sections, one headed happy events and the other headed sad events, as a starting point. Surprisingly many depressed patients leave the sad side blank, refusing to acknowledge unhappiness in their lives. It is important to allow adequate time for the patient to explain to the group what he has either drawn or written. The patients', not he therapist's, interpretation is what counts. Discussion of the work with group members is of great value.

Secondly, art can be used for its social value as an activity in collage and making seasonal decorations. Thirdly, art can be a most valuable hobby, allowing self expression, creativity and a means of social involvement through art club membership, classes and painting holidays, possibly preventing recurrence of a depressive illness. For example, Mrs. F. is now an active member of her local community, having benefitted greatly from day hospital treatment, she now has a full satisfying life. She has been given help and support to re-start her interest in painting, patchwork and cooking, and in coming to terms with her problems and taking the next step in her rehabilitation. Her cane has badges representing the many countries she has visited. She even managed to fly to Tenerife to visit her brother.

THE NEXT STEP

The next step refers to the rehabilitation link between day hospital discharge and community integration of functional psychogeriatric patients with a diagnosis of depression. This can be realized through the formation of self help groups that meet once a week either in each others' homes or on outings together. The formation of such groups revolves around the therapeutic value and healing power of friendship and caring. These few lines were used within the hospital psychotherapeutic group prior to this self help group's formation:

> A FRIEND IS ONE TO WHOM ONE MAY POUR OUT ALL THE CONTENTS OF ONE'S HEART, CHAFF AND GRAIN TOGETHER, KNOWING THAT THE GENTLEST OF HANDS WILL TAKE IT AND SIFT IT, KEEP WHAT IS WORTH KEEPING AND WITH A BREATH OF KINDNESS BLOW THE REST AWAY.

Aims of Self Help Groups

The idea of forming self help groups arose out of the need to maintain the level of function achieved by attendance at the day hospital and by monitoring any psychological, physical and social changes, to prevent hospital re-admission. Some patients were in danger of becoming too dependent on the day hospital structure, fearsome of discharge and unable to maintain themselves in the community. To prevent this yo-yo effect of re-admissions, it seemed a logical step to form a day hospital-community link, thus taking the next step in their rehabilitation programme. Since re-admission to hospital reinforces their idea of failure, surely prevention must represent success.

Formation of Link Groups

Phased discharge was used to wean the patients off the day hospital gradually, by reducing their days of attendance until they were only attending once fortnightly. The nucleus of the community group was an extension of the relationships built up during the course of the small psychotherapeutic feelings group. The hospital and community groups ran concurrently until a team decision was taken to discharge the patient and to follow-up in the community self help group. A consultant psychiatrist made periodic visits to the groups. His interest, support and seal of approval set these groups on a firm basis.

Rehabilitation Concepts

The rehabilitation concepts were:

1. To strengthen and develop relationships among people who share similar problems within the day hospital setting.
2. To supply motivation to return to former levels of independence.

The model for the original community group was taken from the author's own personal experience. The author's mother suffered a reactive depression following her husband's death. An extremely loving couple, my mother thought she could not live without her husband. Most of her friends were also widowed and by caring for each other, sharing interests, and giving each other support she was helped through this sad experience and is now leading a well adjusted active life.

The ladies in the community link group lacked the motivation which the healthy ladies were fortunate enough to have. By helping to supply that missing link having the group meet

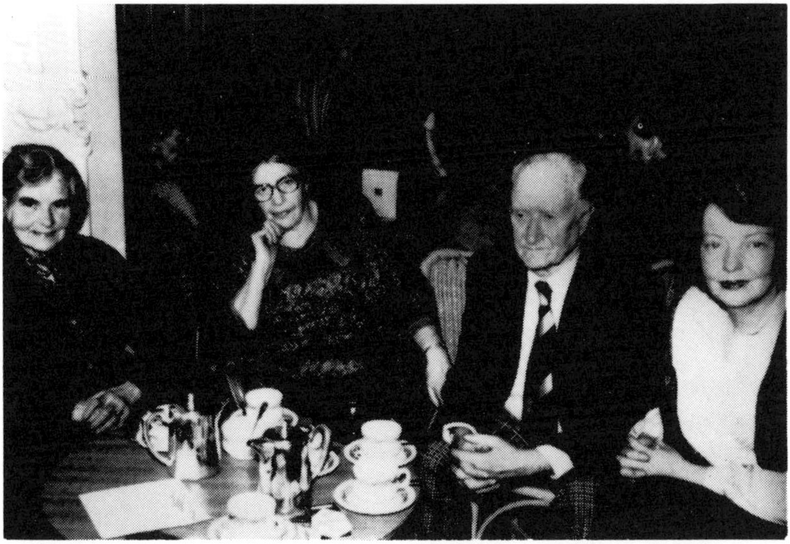

Enjoying Tea Together

weekly in each other's homes, the motivation to resume daily living activities would be strengthened. There is nothing like expecting visitors to make you get on with household chores.

Most of the people had completely lost confidence and interest in socialising, thus making themselves prisoners in their own homes. To break this habit and provide motivation apart from meeting in each other's homes, outings were arranged every third week and, where appropriate, interests and community involvement developed.

The Therapist's Role

The therapist's function as co-ordinator of the group is:

1. Acting as confidant and friend, to supply, as appropriate, support, affection and humour, to help the ladies work out the solutions to their problems and to encourage them to nourish one another.
2. Giving support without taking away independence and withdrawing support at the appropriate time.

3. Acting as a catalyst and endeavoring to give insight and modify behaviour in a way that evolves naturally and is nonthreatening.
4. Suppling enthusiasm and imagination as these ingredients are infectious.
5. Monitoring progress, giving feedback to the hospital and intervening when necessary, thus creating a feeling of security, stability and caring.

Criteria for Selection

In order to be eligible for the group a participant needed to reside in the geographical area, have minimal family support and be living alone. All but one person in the original group met these criteria. One member lived with her husband but suffered great marital disharmony due to his drinking problem. She developed cancer and and the group supported her until her death in a hospice one year later. The group still keeps in touch with her husband, now a frail old man who suffers great pangs of guilt and sadness.

Caring and Sharing

Since this is a self help group concept, caring and sharing amongst each other is the most important function of the group and the one that is largely responsible for the group's success. The little everyday transactions cement friendship, give pleasure and help alleviate feelings of despair and isolation. The following brief examples illustrate the breadth of activities that can be used for facilitating re-entry into the community.

Last year's Christmas outing was held at a very select golf club due to the generosity of the group "Uncle", now a widower with no children whose wife was a patient until her death. The group in turn helped him cope with his loss, particularly at such times as the first anniversary of his wife's death. On the group's first anniversary an outing was planned for a beach picnic. One of the members had been a nanny in this community in her youth. This brought back many happy memories.

A coffee craft shop in a village outside Edinburgh is owned

and run by a former community occupational therapist. Two of the groups meet for the monthly combined get together in this delightful setting. Further examples of caring and sharing are the exchange of telephone numbers among group members and visiting group members in hospital, nursing home and hospice.

Problem Solving

Problems related to everyday living, interpersonal relationships, medication compliance and symptoms of illness are worked out by talking about them, setting targets, and carrying out gradual desensitization programmes in as natural a way as possible. For example, patients with agoraphobia went Christmas shopping to a large department store, and to visit the cinema to see the film *Ghandi.* By using a situation where they were best motivated and by giving quiet confidence and the gentle push which is necessary, fears can be lessened.

Some problems can be solved by discussing them individually, within the group or with the therapist alone. The elderly have many problems that cannot be solved, however; for example, increasing age and frailty, widowhood or financial insecurity, but by using the concept of caring and sharing within the small intimate group, they find it possible to learn to accept what cannot be changed.

Where possible, it is extremely important to include and inform relatives of the group's function and plans, giving support, counselling and intervention when necessary.

RESULTS

Nearly three years later, bonds have been strengthened and members of the groups helped through changing circumstances by its active caring, sharing support and affection.

Success is demonstrated by:

1. The formation of a second successful group one year later, and a third group eighteen months later;
2. High weekly attendance figures;
3. Minimum hospital intervention;

4. Continuing support for frail members requiring residential care and a member requiring hospice care;
5. Strengthened community links leading to an enhanced quality of life.

CONCLUSION

The rehabilitation concepts of strengthening relationships and supplying motivation have been fulfilled; lessons have been learned. The groups have each taken on their separate identities. Due to increasing numbers of elderly, limited facilities and finance, development of such groups could add to enhanced quality of life in a very positive way and so prevent hospital readmission. Gradually handing over the groups to specially chosen volunteers is the next step, thus enabling new groups to be developed.

Perhaps better than in any other way, the therapeutic importance of the group can be demonstrated through the words of Annie:

> *What the group means to me:* The group is my lifeline. Each week I look forward to getting away from the house for a few hours (except when I am entertaining the others in my own home) and it gives me a chance to forget myself in the congenial company of the other members of the group. We exchange needs and views and rejoice when things go well and try to help when they go ill. It all helps to restore one's confidence and makes life worth living.

Treatment of Depression in Institutionalized Older Persons

Ingrid Due Pedersen

Denmark has a population of about five million persons. Of these, about 700,000 are 67 years and older, 167,000 are 80 years and older and 27,000 are 90 years and older. Six percent of the elderly over 67 years are in nursing homes. Thirty three percent of the elderly over 80 are in nursing homes. Characteristic of this century is the phenomenon that the population of elderly has increased, particularly the very elderly or those over 80 years. The purpose of this paper is to describe programming for the elderly in Denmark with a focus on illustrating treatment concepts using examples of occupational therapy in a nursing home. Elderly policy in Denmark is designed to allow the elderly to live in their own houses or apartments as long as possible. This means that the government offers the old people support such as:

—visiting nurse in the home
—a home health aide to help with cleaning, shopping, dressing, toileting*
—meals on wheels
—activities provided in the home if the person is unable to attend a day care center
—transportation to a day care center
—transportation to and from a day nursing home, where care and treatment are available

---

Based on a presentation at the International Symposium: Occupational Therapy Approaches to Depression in Older Adults, Pre-Congress Conference, XIII International Congress of Gerontology, July, 1985, Columbia University, New York.

*In Denmark these persons are less specialized than the American home health aides. Danish aides provide any needed assistance.

When you offer these opportunities it is possible for old people to stay at home, even those with a great need for care. These policies have positive as well as negative aspects. It should not be necessary to tell about the positives but I would like to mention two of the negatives which are important for the nursing homes. Many of the elderly (in fact most of them) get very lonely due to a loss of friends and the fact that family members are old themselves. Living alone without any other contact than a home health aide for a daily visit results in the precipitation of a senile dementia either in its early phase or a reawakening of a long dormant problem. Many of these old people are also living with depression or other mental disorders. The treatment of these mental disorders in older people has previously not been prevalent in Denmark. But this has changed and today both family doctors and other members of the medical profession are more alert to the symptoms and older persons receive better treatment for these depressions.

It is very difficult to distinguish between depression and senile dementia when a person has been living with both for a long time without getting any treatment. As a result old people who are in nursing homes today and will be there during the nest years are a very difficult group both physically and mentally.

NURSING HOMES IN DENMARK

The nursing home used as a model for this discussion has 49 old people. During the last three years we have used mental stimulation as a treatment for those who have both depression and senile dementia. The mental stimulation is provided primarily in the occupational therapy department but the whole staff is learning about mental stimulation as well.

In addition to the medical treatment, a subject which I shall not touch here, there are features which are of great importance in their treatment. Usually, the elderly have fixed ideas or assumptions, habits and attitudes from their earlier lives. Or, in other words, the older persons are individually influenced by the changes in physical, emotional and social age, by traits developed during a long life through familiar human contacts, and by hard earned experiences from life as well as by various personal experiences.

ROLE OF THERAPISTS

A needed condition for the therapists and other members of the staff is perceptive insight into all these factors in order to give the individual patient the appropriate treatment. From the beginning you must try to gain the old person's confidence, establish good personal contact, and little by little gather pieces of information about the old person's earlier life. It is important for the person to be able to freely express their thoughts without feeling forced. Other staff also receive valuable information about the patient's earlier life related to social and disease conditions that they must record. In this way all staff can benefit from the information and prevent the older person from having to answer the same questions over and over again. Such information shows a distinct yet comprehensive diagnostic profile and helps to provide a fruitful basis for treatment. Good treatment must be built on each person's individual condition. It is far easier, and much more important, to activate the older patient in doing something which has had his/her interest earlier in life, even very long ago.

In order to evaluate the underlying reasons for the older person's debilitated condition, it is necessary to get an impression of the extent of the changes due to increasing age. An in-depth familiarity with the person's physical and sensory status and habit patterns will allow the therapist to capitalize on periods of optimal well being as well as deviations from habitual performance.

The ultimate goal must be to divert the older person from his/her disease and from sad subjects. Every kind of activity, dresssing, cooking, nature and other areas of earlier interest are potentially positive sources of involvement. In addition to this, efforts must be made to have the older person accept that his/her life must go on under the new and possibly limited conditions.

ROLE OF THE FAMILY

The family is an important source of cooperation in this work. Often the family is able to give pieces of information about the older person's earlier life, information of importance to treatment. The contact between the family and the older person is also important. The relationship must be preserved during a close, safe, warm contact be it with earlier comfortable objects or the comfort gained from holding hands and having a quiet talk.

CONTACT PERSON

A unique quality of our program is the use of the contact person. The nursing home assigns one member of the staff to every old person. This contact person follows the older person from the first visit in his/her home before moving into the nursing home, assists together with the family during the moving in and continues to be available during the first difficult days in the nursing home. The contact person will be that member of the staff who has the closest contact with the old person during their stay at the nursing home. This person is very important in treatment.

Older persons require that treatment and instruction be given to them in accordance with their individual ability. Therefore it is important that all staff have knowledge of the special teaching approaches useful with the elderly.

SPEED

Old people are slower in their reactions, it is more difficult to perceive the signals that come to the brain and it also takes longer to react appropriately. This means that instructions should be given slowly to allow the older person time to integrate each concept, to motor plan and to process the information. Even a little variation in the learning tempo means a disproportionate increase in troubles for the older person. Situations in which older persons feel stress because of the speed must be avoided, and instruction arranged so the older person can select the speed. In long term planning it is important to calculate sufficient timc for repetition during training. Using short periods of instruction and many pauses in which the information can have time to settle are important considerations.

NOISE

Older persons have problems when many signals come to the brain at the same time and need to be processed. This is demonstrated in the so called “coffee party effect”. Probably everyone has noticed that it is difficult for older persons to attend to the conversations going on across a table. In such cases older persons often choose to keep out of the conversation. Usually it is not because they are not interested, knowledgeable or able, but because the conversation takes place under conditions which are disadvantageous for the process of abstract thinking by the older person. On the contrary, if the conversation is held under suitable conditions, meaning that irrelevant noise is reduced as much as possible, and the speed is suitably slow, you will see that the older person can take part brilliantly. Perhaps you will find that the elderly can come up with rather important contributions with their life experience as background.

Group work/group discussions ought to be practised frequently in work with the elderly. But there must be a fixed structure in the work. Discussions and conversations in the group are managed in such a way that no one speaks when a discussion is underway and so that one person is allowed to finish before the next starts to speak. Often main points must be summed up and stressed. The planning of the group work must be followed by precise rules as to how the course should be structured.

SIGHT

The senses are weakened with increasing years, especially sight and hearing. Older people need more light than younger people, both common lighting and direct lighting. An extra lamp with direct light on the working place is an important help but care must be taken that there is no glare. Quick shifts in the strength of the light must be avoided as it is difficult for the elderly to adapt to it. If quick shifts are unavoidable the elderly must be given time to adapt to them. A well lighted work place is a good thing, but the common lighting of the room must not be so weak that it demands too much adaptation on the part of the elderly person. Turning the light on and off often, as with slides, makes the instruction less effective as the eye cannot readily accommodate to the adaptation process. It also takes older persons longer to focus and fixate on details of pictures, diagrams and drawings in his/her mind. Therefore, more time is needed just to watch. The picture ought to be shown on the screen for a longer time, and you must emphasize the important things in the picture. Older persons also have difficulty distinguishing shades of colours, especially blue-violet colours. Red and yellow should be used when something must be thrown in relief.

HEARING

Hearing is weakened with increasing age. High notes are difficult to hear and background noise can be distracting. Acoustics must be watched, as for instance noise from the street, music and speech that are not a part of the immediate situation. You must speak loud and clear with pauses and you must place yourself in such a way that the older person can see you when you are speaking.

MEMORY

Everyone recognizes that the memory of older persons is no longer what it was. The fact is, the older person's problem is not so much to retain what they have learned as, to a greater extent, to retrieve thoughts when they are needed. This means that it is important to make sure the older person receives some clear signals to call upon when necessary. As an example, it is difficult for older persons to recall longer instructions when doing an activity. A note fastened to the loom with a few short and clear catchwords can help.

MOTIVATION

It is important not only to create a relaxed atmosphere but also to create a climate conducive to motivation. In our nursing home we are using mental stimulation to treat old people. The two groups we are working with will be described. One is a music group, in which most nursing home residents participate. The other is a special group for those in whom dementia is advanced. The contact person is very important for the work with these groups. This person gives current information about the residents to the staff working with the groups. After every group meeting, the staff and the contact person discuss what has happened in the group. At this meeting, we have the chance to find out if the elderly are reacting in a way that makes it necessary to take them out of the group and offer them another kind of treatment. This only happened once in the three years of the group's existence. Since we know so much about every old person in the group, it is possible for us to ask questions and obtain answers that alert us to the different kind of depression that might occur to members of the group.

SONG AS STIMULATION

Music stimulation is a method to activate persons suffering from mental disorders. A gold mine of mental stimulation is hidden in every song. Music and song are the means to get in contact, and in spite of the reduction of intellectual functions such as concentration and memory, it is possible to bring musical lacunas to light and to make the most of these for physical and psychological stimulation. To sing the songs of the season not only dealing with the weather, but also nature, the life of birds, animals, plants and trees can give the older person an experience of reality. The contents of the songs are supplemented with pictures and material collected from nature. These recollections can help patients remember the year, the place where they are and the date of their birth. Folksongs and ballads contain references to love, birth, death. Common practise and morality strike and awaken feelings which are expressed through the singing of a familiar song in a familiar melody. One may succeed in getting participants to express their feelings in words in connection with the contents of the songs. The rhythm of the songs can also be used as a most important element. With rhythm instruments (drums, claves, triangles, maracas, etc.) the residents can join in accompaniment to the songs. In addition to concentration this demands a process of memorizing, as everybody must learn to join in correctly with the instruments at the appointed parts in the melody.

The songs must be sung in a suitable key and at a speed which makes it possible for the content of the words to be understood. The accompaniment can be guitar, accordian or another transportable instrument, which allows the leader to walk among the patients to maintain contact with each one. In many cases singing can give expression to feelings or moods which the old person is unable to articulate but whose existence shows in the evident pleasure of singing them.

DANCE AND MOTION

Dance can be used for activation, retraining and maintenance of the body's functions as well as to give and receive feelings and touch in an acceptable manner after a structuralized pattern which is agreed upon. In order not to get tired of dancing it is necessary to warm up the body from a sitting position. With a simple melody the leader will be able to compose the movements to be done and to sing them at the same time. Gradually, the patients will learn to sing the song while they perform the exercises.

To get everybody on the dance floor the opening for the dancing could be stepping to music in different rhythms, holding hands, two and two around the room, finishing in a big circle. Old Danish singing-games can be danced, and the participants instructed in simple folk dances from foreign countries. The session must end with familiar dances, danced with partners, where the most important thing is the recognition and the pleasure in spontaneously being able to dance them. To benefit from the music stimulation the level of function in the group must be fairly homogeneous, keeping the patients' various responses to their emotional handicaps in mind.

THE ROOM

It is important that the room in which the music course takes place be spacious, have bright colours, good acoustics, and that the lighting effects, day light as well as artificial light, be adequate. Light stacking chairs which the older persons themselves can carry are an advantage, as this offers possibilities for easily changing the activities. For instance, being seated around the table then getting into a circle on the floor. Also, it is good for the elderly to move into other surroundings. The walk from the department to the ward and back again can be an experience.

THE BREAK

The break is part of the music stimulation. The coffee and tea drinking in common implies that the table is set, an action many of them have done during their lifetime which now seems to be new and not understandable. The ritual in passing around the sugar, the cream and the tea has the same effect and should be repeated to promote success. Flowers and branches of the season decorate the table, which gives the occasion for repeating the names and creates an awareness of the current season. Sitting together around the table also gives rich opportunities for remembering each other's names and in this way strengthens their identity.

PEDAGOGY

The person having the responsibility for the music stimulation must collect the musical material, be in possession of as much knowledge as possible about the elderly's earlier and present lives and must also prepare his/her individual treatment. The music stimulation is neither entertainment nor lessons. It cannot serve to "kill time". The stimulation should give the person experiences to enrich his present situation. Naturally, one should try to meet the person at his level, which is determined by his emotional difficulty. As in all treatment, respect for the individual is a condition for establishing positive contact.

LOWER FUNCTIONING GROUP

A second group was formed because of the need to compose groups as homogenously as possible. Sex, age and background matters little. The second group consisted of six to seven members who caused problems for the departments. They were residents who could not sit still, who wandered around, made a mess of things, walked into other residents and so forth. These residents needed to be watched over constantly by the staff and could not be mixed in with higher functioning residents.

STAFF

In principle, all staff members can participate; however, we have found it appropriate that this group work take place under the supervision of occupational therapy. A person from therapy participates together with two members from the ward staff. Initially, the nursing staff was thoroughly briefed on the goals and the procedures of mental stimulation, and after consultation they agreed to give this program very high priority.

The contact person for each resident is involved as much as possible.

THE ROOM

It is important that all "the meetings" of the group take place in the same room, and that the room be closed for other activities. It is not possible to hold the attention of the group if too many things are going on in the room at the same time. We have made our arrangements in a room in the basement. This room is used at other times for music and by a reading group. It is advantageous if the room can be comfortably decorated with pillows, chairs, and wall hangings. This makes the group members feel more confident and increases their involvement in the activity.

DETAILS OF A GROUP MEETING

The group meets every day from 10:00 am to 11:30 am and every afternoon from 2:30 pm to 3:30 pm. The members are called by the same person from the department, walk the same route along a red line glued to the floor. They talk about the red line, where it leads, and what they will be doing. The door to the meeting room is also painted red.

Every person has his/her own chair where there is a pillow. Each person has his/her own colour and a similar pillow is placed in the member's own chair in the department.

The meeting begins with coffee and an effort to calm down group members who may be agitated or upset that day. Soon they talk about which song should be sung. Songs are chosen by turns and a new song is sung every time. At least this was our intention, but usually the same two songs are suggested. So these songs are faithfully sung each time and we talk about why we chose this particular song or hymn.

Following this is a period of orientation to time using a large wall calendar. Maximum member participation is encouraged. We also celebrate if it happens to be someone's birthday.

Then begins an orientation to oneself. Staff begins with their own names and each person's name is written in large letters on the blackboard. When all the names are on the board we read them and everyone must remember their own name. Occasionally, someone is able to remember the name of the person sitting next to him/her, but the most important thing is to remember one's own name. Staff question members all the time, especially the noisy persons who must be activated and stimulated by addressing them.

We make a lot out of the seasons. This gives many opportunities for chats and recollection: Christmas, Easter, summer and winter are obviously good subjects.

The day's menu provides an opportunity to talk about recipes and how things are made. Experience has shown that the old people are pleased when we talk about recipes. We write down the recipes even if it is difficult to remember the figures and letters.

Pictures, objects and cooking implements are placed on the table to stimulate a chat. Having these things placed in front of the members makes it easier to talk about them. Old household items such as a wash board for scrubbing laundry, an iron or a yardstick have been especially popular.

We take great pleasure in examining the objects we gather in plastic bags when we go for a walk. We often create collages from the things we gather. Many of the members enjoy seeing the stone or feather they have picked up themselves and glued in the collage.

The group also takes part in preparations for parties in the residence. Decorations are made, napkins are folded and the group entertains with songs. The song is the means we must often turn to if the members are restless. The group is very active and loves to sing, dance and make rhythm.

GENERAL OBSERVATIONS

It is important that the same staff participate in the group. Staff must be able to manage the sometimes tedious day to day routine that rarely changes. Staff must also be able to involve the inactive residents in the activities. Communication in the group is of vital importance for the group to succeed. Staff must use language which everyone is able to understand. Group members need encouragement to speak for themselves and involve themselves with the activities of the group. Older people, like everyone else, need to be appreciated and rewarded. Some of them like to be praised in words, others are happy for a hug or a handshake.

When the morning group meeting is over the whole group walks to the dining room where they set the table. The group, along with the staff participating in the group, eat together.

In general, the physical activities of the group are a good means to calm down members. Thus, we have chosen to gather the group together again in the afternoon for a walk except when the weather is very bad. Two of the members use wheelchairs and it is always another group member who pushes the chair. While we are walking we talk about what we see and gather things in bags for the next day's activities.

SUMMARY

The main purpose of our approach is to enhance the quality of life in the nursing home from physical, psychological and social perspectives, given the older person's intellectual resources. It is important for the older person to regain as much independence as possible in order to strengthen their sense of identity.

Although the program outcome has not been systematically measured we think we have had good results.

For example:

—We don't have elderly sitting inactive in chairs all day.
—We don't have elderly who are a problem for the staff wandering around, making trouble and requiring constant care.
—We don't have elderly who receive large doses of medicine for mental disorders.
—We do have elderly who became better than they were when they entered the home.
—We do have elderly who are happy and able to take part in the other activities of the home.
—We have elderly who are interested in their own self care and take part in dressing and grooming themselves.
—We do have elderly who are no longer a problem for the home because they are involved from 10:00 am to 4:00 pm, and then are tired.

We believe that these results are useful for the older person and the nursing home—and so we go on!

9-91 3
7-92 7
7-93 9
6-94 12
4-95 19
8-96 21
4-99 28
3/00 35